Secrets
OF
Stress-Free
Entertaining

Chris Cooper

CHRIS COOPER

Copyright ©2022 by Chris Cooper
Secrets of Stress-Free Entertaining The Villages Edition
All rights reserved.

No part of this publication may be reproduced, distributed, or transmitted in any form or by any means, including photocopying, recording, or other electronic or mechanical methods, without the prior written permission of the author except in cases of brief quotations embodied in critical articles and reviews. For information, contact the author at www.chriscooperdesign.com

This is a work of non-fiction. Names, characters, places, and incidents are either factual or products of the author's imagination. Any resemblance to actual persons, living or dead, businesses, companies, events, or locales is entirely coincidental.

Edited by Paula F. Howard, A Howard Activity, LLC

Cover design by Bob Hurley at www.impressionsbookdesignservices.com
Interior Design by Linda Hurley at www.impressionsbookdesignservices.com
Photos are Royalty-Free Images

Aha! Press is an imprint of A Howard Activity, LLC

ISBN: 979-8-9860707-1-1   HARDcover – National Edition

ISBN: 979-8-9860707-2-8   SOFTcover - National Edition

PRINTED IN THE UNITED STATES OF AMERICA

Available for purchase on Amazon.com and at TheWritersMall.com

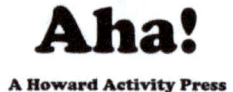

CONTENTS

1
CHAPTER 1
Secrets of Stress-Free Entertaining

9
CHAPTER 2
Let's Make a Plan
10   Party With a Purpose
10   Let's Get Started
13   The Magic of PEAP
16   Gracious Host Protocol
17   Gracious Guest Protocol

21
CHAPTER 3
Week One: Sending Out the Invitation
22   Theme
24   Types of Parties
26   Date
27   Time
27   Guest List
27   Where
29   Menu
29   Budget
30   Master Invitation
31   Summary of Week One

33
CHAPTER 4   PART ONE
Week Two: Making Decisions
33   Fine-Tuning and Deciding on Details
36   Pantry and Refrigerator Basics
40   The Table

43 Baking, Dishes, Prep
46 The Traveling Feast
46 Planning Portions

51
CHAPTER 4   PART TWO
Week Two: Setting the Bar
52 Bring Your Own Bottle (BYOB) Party
52 Where to Place the Bar
52 Storage
53 Barware
54 Stocking the Bar
57 Wine Basics
59 Tips for Pairing Wine with Food
61 **Summary of Week Two**

63
CHAPTER 5   PART ONE
Week Three: Getting It Under Control
63 Final Details
67 Sample Menus
72 Let's Talk About Cheese!
77 The Essential Gougéres
79 The Importance of Tabletop Tents

81
CHAPTER 5   PART TWO
Week Three: All About Templates
81 The Master Template
84 How to Use the Master Template
85 Let's Get Some Practice with the Templates.
87 Practice Template Exercise
91 **Summary of Week Three**

93
CHAPTER 6
Week Four: Almost Party Time
- **93** The Final Countdown
- **101** How to Handle Hiccups
- **102** The Party's Over
- **103** **Summary of Week Four**

105
CHAPTER 7
Favorite Party Recipes
- **105** Brunch
- **109** Appetizers
- **113** Regional Favorites
- **117** Dips
- **120** Cheese
- **123** Salads
- **127** Main Dishes
- **132** Potatoes
- **135** Desserts

143
CHAPTER 8
- **143** **Entertaining is Magical**
- **147** **APPENDIX 1** Holiday Theme Parties
- **153** **APPENDIX 2** Signature Punch Recipes
- **161** **APPENDIX 3** National Party Days
- **175** **APPENDIX 4** Measurements, Substitutions, Cooking Terms
- **181** **APPENDIX 5** Stain Guide
- **185** **APPENDIX 6** Overnight Guests
- **189** **APPENDIX 7** A Glossary of Cheeses
- **197** Recommended Reading
- **199** About the Author

CHRIS COOPER

DEDICATION

This book is dedicated to my Mother, Ethel Cooper, who taught me all the important things like love, friendship, gracious entertaining, and hard work.

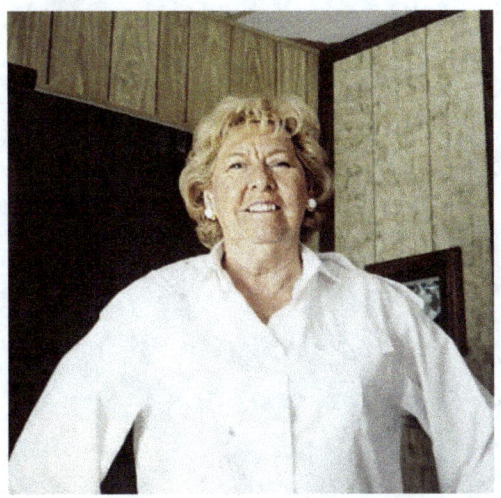

She shared her passions and knowledge from her heart. She had such a hunger for learning and enjoyed a lifetime of creativity and adventure. She genuinely cared for people and had many friends and admirers along the way.

Mom loved living in The Villages, Florida, and she belonged to many clubs setting up their events, dinners, and parties. She absolutely loved to dance! She would often gauge the success of parties that she went to by the amount of dancing she did. I always called her the "Dancing Queen."

Mom was a victim of Covid in January 2020, at the age of 93. At the time of her death, she was planning her "We're back to normal!" party for the time when life would return to normal, after Covid. She thought that would be a time for everyone to celebrate and embrace each other like never before.

I hope this book honors her memory. I know she would have encouraged me to write it.

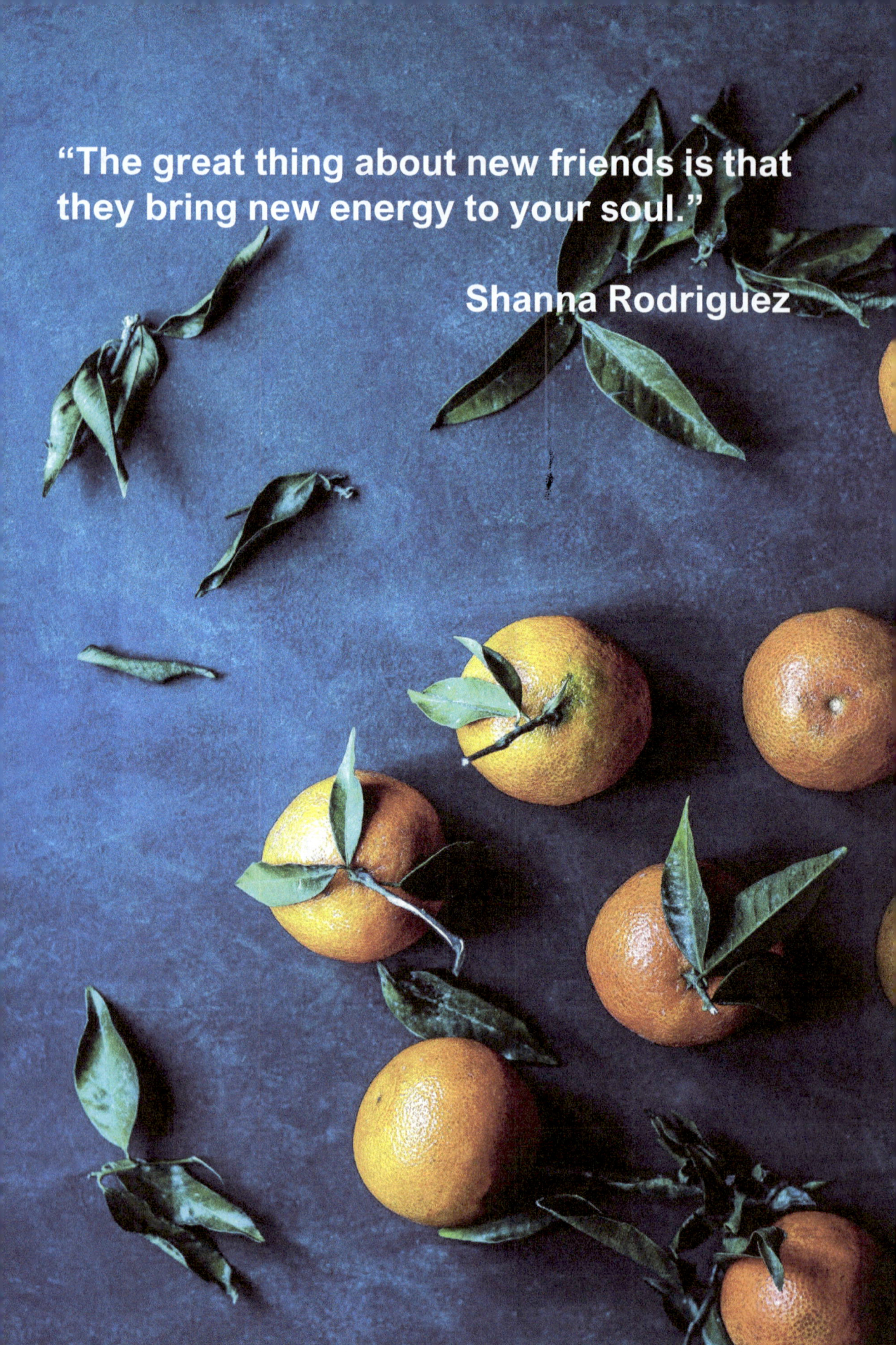

"The great thing about new friends is that they bring new energy to your soul."

Shanna Rodriguez

Chapter One
Secrets of Stress-Free Entertaining

Some may think "stress-free entertaining" is an oxymoron. Does your heart sink at the thought of entertaining? Do you feel dread, panic, or even anxiety? Perhaps you think: "Where do I start?" If this is your response, then I am so glad you chose this book. YES! It is possible to enjoy your own party OF ANY SIZE with both grace and style.

Once you follow the road map in the pages of this book and master the steps, you will gain the important confidence that at will allow you to enjoy your own entertaining events.

An amazing, memorable party is a wonderful combination of art and science. The artistry is in choosing a theme and concept, the beautiful table linens, and decorations. This book is more about the science of putting it all together, and that is what event planning is all about. The real secret of a successful party is a direct result of extraordinary event planning.

This is a book about successful and memorable event planning.

This book will provide you with the tools you need to effortlessly pull together the planning you need to create extraordinary, exciting, and memorable events. I have been successfully teaching these techniques in my classes for years, and my students have continually inspired me with their creativity and enthusiasm. I would like to awaken your inspiration with a step-by-step plan for creating parties that will be enjoyed and remembered. My classes are an hour and a half long every Friday over the course of four weeks which is the ideal amount of time to plan an awesome party. So, let's begin a four-week journey planning every detail of your creation from the initial concept to a successful event.

This book is meant to be interactive, and I hope you will use it as a workbook. I invite you to go through the four-week plan with the goal of either having your own party soon or planning an imagined one in the future. Completing this exercise, and making it personal, will help increase your skills. Entertaining confidently and stress-free, and actually enjoying your own parties, will become easy and fun! Once you master the steps, you'll be capable of throwing together something wonderful with just a few hours' notice. It happens. And you'll be ready.

I have found that those who enjoy entertaining are extremely generous people. They love to give of their time, which is the most precious thing anyone can give. Party-givers love to please, surprise, impress, excite, and inspire. It can be very satisfying to delight the people you care about by giving them of your time and efforts.

In your past, you may have entertained a great deal. Or perhaps you have only hosted family and holiday gatherings. You may be a gourmet chef, and love to cook as I do, or you may hate to cook, and the kitchen is a foreign place to you. Grocery store party platters may be what you choose to serve at your parties. Everyone has their own relationship with their kitchen! While this book has some tried and true recipes which you are encouraged to try, this book is NOT about how skilled of a cook you need to be.

The kitchen has always been my happy place. Cooking and baking for people I love and care about has always been my way of showing them how much they mean to me. It's an integral part of who I am. My best memories involve spending time celebrating with family and friends. Among my treasure trove are memories of waking up on Sunday morning and finding my son's basketball team at the table waiting for my favorite French toast or making thirteen lasagnas for the football team. For me, cooking has always been a source of joy.

I now live alone and get the urge to have some fun in the kitchen. If I ate everything I cooked, it would not have a happy ending. I love to bake cupcakes! Most recipes plan for two dozen cupcakes, and I have to share! I often deliver them anonymously to my neighbors around dessert time. Or I have left some in a pretty box in the driveway on trash collection day. I sometimes deliver banana bread to the doorstep of friends on Easter morning.

Having a special surprise for your postal worker or delivery person is always fun. Their smiles make my day!

For the past few years, I have enjoyed teaching "Entertaining with Grace and Style" at The Enrichment Academy in The Villages, Florida. I've met many creative, inspiring, wonderful residents of The Villages, most of whom are retired. Not wanting to feel stress or anxiety in party planning is a common reason for taking my class. It's normal to feel some anxiety while planning a party, especially when you may not know the people very well, or if you don't have a plan. I will teach you how to have a plan.

*Being able to entertain stress-free
and being able to actually ENJOY your own party
is the ultimate goal.*

The systems and information about event planning detailed in this book are steps I learned from my mother. We lived in the San Francisco Bay Area. Her passion was cooking, and she started a catering business. When it became too busy, she asked me to join her. We mainly catered weddings, just usually not high society events, and we were not gourmet chefs. We made tasty, fresh, recognizable food that people loved. Our menus at times included ham, lasagna, and lots of yummy salads. Usually, it was a buffet, and we elevated everything with our presentation.

Presentation is everything!

Our table settings were always thoughtful with beautiful table linens and draping. Our centerpieces would always receive a "Wow!" We searched for beautiful trays, bowls, and serve ware to create displays that made any bride proud. Our reputation grew and we became extremely busy. I remember cooking for eight different events over a three-day period. And we did it all out of our own home kitchens.

My mother and father eventually retired and moved away, and the business was retired as well. I earned my real estate license and began showing properties. It wasn't long before I realized that in order to get the biggest turnouts to my real estate listings, I needed to make it an "event." During those years there might be fifty homes listed on a Tuesday real estate agent tour. Well, food attracts people and I found that real estate agents were not immune to that logic. So, my events always had food with a theme, something special to make them stop at my listings. My catering background came in handy. Sometimes, we planned an Italian lunch; one hot summer day, we even did a milkshake party. It was important that we planned something different and unexpected, and it seemed to work out beautifully.

My last position was as Vice President and Director of Training for Prudential Insurance Company. That's where I began passing along the secrets of effective event planning to my students.

Then I started my Home Staging Business. I was a pioneer in a brand-new industry. Home staging was, and still is, a way to present what you are selling in the best light possible. As with catering, presentation is everything! It is so important for photographs and video tours to be done well because they are now seen on the Internet. Back then, we began staging events for my home staging business. We grew very quickly expanding to eighteen employees and staging up to fifty homes a month.

One of our largest events was for the launch of our own website. I rented the local Tesla car showroom. It was their first showroom when Tesla was just starting out. We had also changed our logo, so we wrapped our five staging trucks with our name and new logo while having everyone dressed in new uniforms. It was a red-carpet event on a busy street at a time everyone was getting off work. We had photographers acting as paparazzi taking pictures of our 300 guests as they walked up the red carpet. We brought in sofas, tables, chairs, and had television screens continuously showing our website which were showing the videos we had been taking. My mother and I made all the food. Needless to say, we created quite a traffic jam! It was wonderfully received, and business soared as a result.

Then, in 2017, I sold my business and moved to Florida. Since then, I have enjoyed teaching the skills my mother taught me years ago. I learned to enjoy the excitement and joy of entertaining that she shared with me from an early age. Christmas Eve was always her special "Party of the Year." She would start planning for it in July and would begin enjoying the excitement and anticipation months before the event. I used to tease her about doing that.

Entertaining has a long and interesting history. Throughout the world, deals and alliances have been made over cocktails and appetizers for the past several hundred years. Prestige, wealth, and relevance were often dictated by which parties one attended. Those entertainers who planned and staged such parties were under a great deal of pressure from the guest lists to the quality of food and alcohol. They became well known for their skills in assembling every detail since their social status was on the line.

Of course, much has changed, and the most common party now is more casual. But the same customs of gracious entertaining have never gone away. Here, you will be provided with ideas for creating memorable parties that your friends will look forward to attending and remember long after the event is over.

This book is being written after we have all suffered through a difficult time of Covid-19. There has been a great deal of pain, sacrifice, and loss, including my own mother who I lost in 2020. I believe the pandemic has only amplified how important our connections are with those whom we truly care about. Our memories are especially important.

One of the hardest parts of the pandemic was the isolation, so our memories from the past have become very precious. Connections, interactions, and touching were restricted to a video screen. For those of us who are "huggers," there was a true sense of loss.

As we turn the corner and emerge from the time of Covid-19, entertaining and sharing with our friends and family has become more important than ever in re-establishing those connections again. We are all looking forward to enjoying events and participating in gatherings as we return to a normalcy that we used to take for granted. It is time to open our doors once more and begin participating and celebrating life again. Yes, it is time to make new memories!

Because this book is designed to be a valuable reference and resource for you, I have included practical, useful information such as ingredient substitutions, pantry and refrigerator basics, supplies and tools, basic bar setup, and wine basics.

The most important components of effective event planning are the two-page master templates explained in Week Three of our learning system. These templates will crystalize your concept, aid in menu planning, and allow you to evaluate and adjust your menu details as needed. Learning to use the templates is a vital step to bringing it all into focus for you. These systems will guide you through planning, focusing on key details, and helping to build the confidence which allows you to enjoy your own party.

No matter what your background, this book will teach you the skills needed to gain the confidence to plan a wonderful party. A successful party is the result of good event planning. Having a road map for every detail of your party is the secret to creating a memorable event.

Because enjoying a meal with friends and family is so important to our mental and physical health, I would suggest getting into a celebratory mood beginning with making every day, every meal . . . special. Even if you are alone! Take the time to make something good and healthy for yourself. Start paying attention to your own diet. Try new recipes. Turn on your favorite music as you slice and dice. Use your best china . . . every day! Why not? It's meant to be used and enjoyed. Buy cloth napkins and some pretty glasses. How about a new table runner and placemats? Get them in colors that you love, and which make you happy.

Every day should be a celebration and a time to appreciate and be grateful. Food is an integral part of life and that which keeps us healthy and strong. Sharing with others is the garnish that makes it all worthwhile!

SECRETS OF STRESS-FREE ENTERTAINING

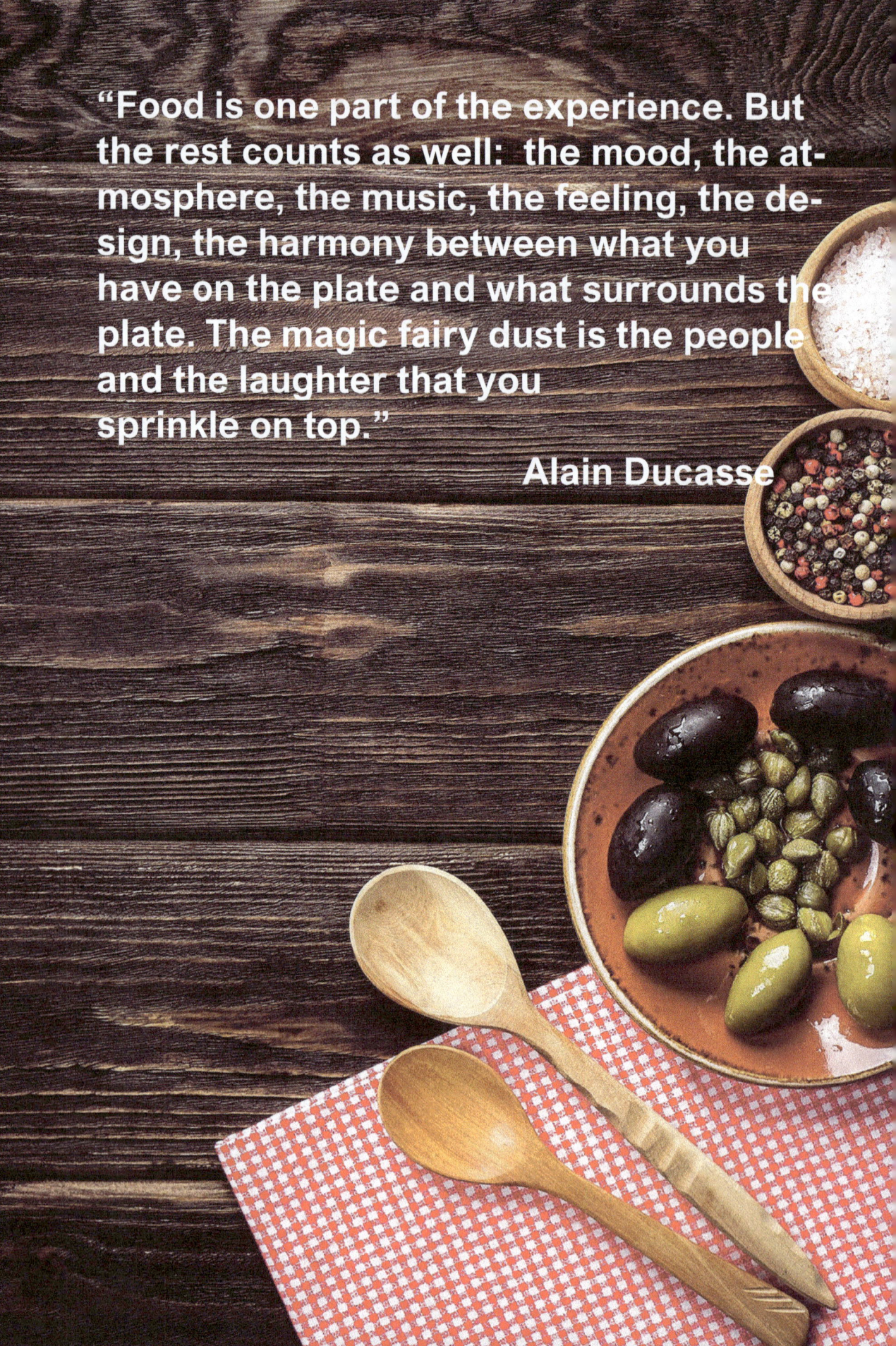

"Food is one part of the experience. But the rest counts as well: the mood, the atmosphere, the music, the feeling, the design, the harmony between what you have on the plate and what surrounds the plate. The magic fairy dust is the people and the laughter that you sprinkle on top."

— Alain Ducasse

Chapter 2
Let's Make a Plan

There is no mystery in planning a party that rocks!
But there are secrets that will make you a party magician!

Stress-free entertaining is having a plan and preparation is EVERYTHING! The terms "event" and "party" will be used interchangeably throughout this book. Every party should be an event, large or small. **The size of your party is of no consequence.** This special event planning system will prepare you for a cozy dinner party for two or a gala for three hundred guests.

Four weeks is the ideal amount of time to prepare for your event. Our four-week template is the ideal way to start your entertaining journey. It gives you the right amount of time to plan everything down to the last detail. Once you have all the details under control, you can truly enjoy your guests and your own party. By mastering the four-week plan, you can easily adapt and prepare for whatever is thrown at you, whether it's in the future or as close as tonight!

You may be single, or you may be living with a partner. I encourage you to talk over plans with your partner; have fun with it! Working as a team, you can easily divide the preparation needs and enjoy the party together!

PARTY WITH A PURPOSE!

One bonus you can incorporate into your parties is to "Party with a Purpose"! Be a leader and create a "giving" community. If you can gather for one reason, why not two? Think how special that would make your party:

- Obtain a list of families in need of holiday foods and/or gifts. You could get a direction and some names from local churches or social service agencies. Adopt those families either as a group or, if your neighbors are willing, one family could adopt another family.
- Obtain a list of local families that would appreciate a Christmas tree delivered complete with lights and decorations.
- Help some of the elderly in the neighborhood put up their own holiday decorations. You can all have a party after the hard work is finished, then another party in January when you help take the decorations down.
- Create holiday baskets for the local food pantry.

Parties with a purpose don't need to be limited to the holidays. A party in August could include gathering school supplies for local schools. Around Mother's Day, imagine the smiles if you brought flowers to forgotten mothers in nursing facilities. What about a cookie-making party or cookie exchange? If everyone made or brought a double batch of their favorite cookie recipe you could enjoy the party, then deliver some to First Responders, Urgent Care Centers, or a local hospital. There are so many ways to have a party and spread joy beyond the event. Having a meaningful purpose for your party will leave a warm memory for everyone who attends.

LET'S GET STARTED!

To begin, put together your own party planning binder. This will include all your ideas, plans, recipes, and strategies. It's your own idea book for future parties. You can divide it into different categories: Ideas, guest lists, recipes, past parties, and more.

Week three of our plan (Chapter 5) offers a Master Template which I encourage you to use for every party. Keep your completed template inside your binder either under 'References" or "Past Parties." You can even categorize it as "Next Parties." You get the idea. In your binder, record every party that you plan. This includes ideas, pictures, what went right, what went wrong, what was served, what you wore, and who you invited. You'll be glad you did.

Get in the habit of pulling recipes. If you see something in a magazine you like, pull it out on the spot! Don't tell yourself you will find it later. You won't. Even if you don't think you'll use the recipe in the future, but you like it, that's a decision for later. You may use that recipe as a spark of inspiration. Below are some publications which might inspire you:

Food and Wine Magazine	Better Homes and Garden
Taste of Home	Bon Appetit
Food Network	Martha Stewart Living
Eating Well	Good Housekeeping
Woman's Day	Veranda

Remember, some people have dietary restrictions, with Diabetes being a concern for many. The publication, **Diabetes Self-Management,** offers healthy recipes and ideas. Gluten-free, Keto, Vegan, and Vegetarian diets all have guidelines you may wish to incorporate into your menu planning.

One rule is to never serve a dish before you have tried it first. Don't serve dishes you don't personally like! For instance, you may feel that your guests expect a seafood choice—maybe shrimp. But you are allergic to shellfish (many people are.) If you serve too much and have leftovers, it's not something you will eat. Serve only items for which you will be grateful there are leftovers to enjoy. Or you could purposely make too much and make sure you have leftovers!

In your binder, include pictures of pretty table settings, centerpieces, and party ideas. This is your own personal Idea Book reflecting on what you like and the type of entertaining you want to do. Update it as a living book as you go along.

Become a student of parties. When you go to other parties, watch what works and what doesn't work. I'm not saying to be judgmental, but view everything as a learning experience. Was there enough seating? Enough food? What foods were guests drawn to? How was it presented? What could have been improved? Take it all in! How did it flow? Was there a bottleneck at the bar area? Was there a place to stow your purse or wrap? Were there enough trash cans? If you see something you liked, don't hesitate to copy it! Copying something is your biggest compliment! If there is a dish you love, ask for the recipe. Most hosts are happy to share them and it's a great way to make a new friend.

Presentation is everything.

The goal of entertaining is showing people that you care down to the smallest details. Time is the most precious commodity you can give and demonstrates how much you care. The way you present the food will make your event memorable. You may not be a master chef but being a master of presenting a lovely display will surprise and delight your guests. Anticipate their needs and I guarantee you will derive incredible joy just from seeing their pleasure.

This book includes many easy, tried-and-true recipes. You may not have time to try all of them, you may not even want anything to do with the kitchen. But you can still be a master entertainer, even if you get all your food from a restaurant or simply buy party platters from your favorite grocery store. In fact, I encourage you to be familiar with what's available in case you need to rely on local sources in a pinch.

Here is the secret to a fantastic party: Presentation. Don't put food on the table in the same containers that you picked up at the store. Re-plate everything using beautiful dishes or platters. I have one friend who puts everything on the party table with plastic tops of containers still bearing their price tags! Never do that. Display the food, perhaps dress it up with surrounding greenery like some parsley. Elevate it! The various angles of dishes add a dramatic, pleasing effect. Then, take the store containers and bury them in the trash. No one will know that you didn't spend all day in the kitchen. (Unless you tell them.)

THE MAGIC OF PEAP

I recently read an article reflecting on entertaining in the decades of the 50's and 60's. Funny, but I don't believe modern-day entertaining needs to be much different. There are valuable traditions with grace and civility that add to being a gracious guest or host. For instance, the article cited parties of old having expectations and certain steps in the process of entertaining such as putting name tags on your table indicating where people should sit. That's not a bad thing. Would you like some of your favorite friends to meet? Sit them next to each other. Do you know that two of your friends don't really get along, or have anything in common? Put them at opposite ends of the table.

Today, however, invitations may be sent electronically through emails, texts, or Evite. In most cases, I still prefer a handwritten invitation. Why? Because it is unexpected these days which makes an invitation in the mail stand out; it becomes special. Whichever you choose to do, the goal is the same. We always want our guests to enjoy the time spent together.

Remember, the objective of any event is to make it memorable. Who wants to throw a ho-hum party? Below are components for a successful party:

Make lots of lists.
Keep them together and organized.

Preparation

Have you ever noticed preparation for anything gives it a better outcome? That is the key to stress-free entertaining. This book will help you know which lists to make, how to manage your time, what tools you'll need, and how to plan for any event. Making lists will save your sanity!

Expectations

Creating and exceeding expectations is the goal. Your techniques and party planning skills can help elevate those expectations. Yours will be the parties everyone looks forward to attending.

Anticipation

Anticipation begins with your planning and extends to the invitation. That is another reason I prefer a handwritten invitation. The invitation should communicate excitement about what's coming by telling them about what is planned. Anticipation is most easily created by the theme you choose. What is the purpose for your party? What is going to make it different than other parties? Remember, you create the excitement.

Presentation

The way things look is everything! It's called "presentation." I encourage you to appeal to all five senses in creating the magic that makes an event very special and one to remember.

Sights and Smells

This does not relate to cost and is not difficult. It only has to be planned and executed well. A successful presentation appeals to all the senses.

Sight—Create that excitement as they come through the door. Clean up and hose down the front porch, plant some new flowers, have a pretty front door. Make it welcoming. Hang a wreath. If it is the rainy season, have a place for umbrellas and wet jackets. Have your party ready to begin the moment your guests walk through the door.

Smell—Have something wonderful cooking. Don't cook fish or curry the night before. Nor do you want something that smells like perfume or sweet air fresheners. Many people have allergies. Use a lemon, cinnamon, apple, and orange scents which are all pleasant and natural.

Appealing to the Sense of Smell

It's important to appeal to all the senses. Having this combination simmering on the stove will make your entire house smell like the holidays. This will definitely add another layer and important detail in your successful event.

> **Christmas Simmer**
>
> 1/8 cup dried orange peel
> 3 cinnamon sticks
> 10 cloves
> 1/2 tsp caraway seeds
> 4 bay leaves
> 1/2 tbsp. whole allspice
> 1 tsp. coriander seeds
> 1/2 tsp. dill seeds
>
> Cook in 2 cups of water on top of stove. Bring to a boil and then reduce to a simmer for an hour or so. Watch that the water does not boil away. Can be saved in a jar, refrigerated, and reheated several times during the season.

Sound

Take some care with a playlist even if you enlist some help. Have the volume low enough to enable conversation, but loud enough to set the tone. Let the type of party dictate what music you choose. Having an Octoberfest party? Get some German music! A luau? Some soft Hawaiian music would be nice. Once you define the reason for your party, the easier this decision will become.

Taste

Have your bar area set up and ready to go. Have some nuts, candy, or light appetizers set out when people arrive.

Touch

This is one sense that is often overlooked. Textural napkins or interesting napkin rings can add to the experience. Also, handing out small token gifts to take home after the party adds to the memories.

It's all in the details!

Be intuitive to your guests' needs. Anticipate how the party will flow. Where will people put their purses and coats? Where will people put their trash? How will the traffic flow?

If you have the luxury of four weeks to plan your party, you will have lots of time to insert the important details that make your party special and memorable. The greatest compliment you can receive is for people to remember your event long after the date.

Planning Ahead
If you plan on doing lots of entertaining, do some planning when you arrange the furniture in your home. Make sure you have enough seating for the size of group. I have found ottomans a great source for additional seating. Tuck them into corners or under tables when not in use. Have a stash of folding chairs in the garage or spare closet.

Make sure to remove cords or flimsy rugs so people won't trip. Arrange the room for an easy flow. Keep in mind where you place your bar. Adding leaves to dining tables may be a good choice.

Activities
In your party planning, try to incorporate a place for activities. We are all still kids at heart and everyone loves to play! If you are a karaoke crowd, leave room for equipment. Dancing is an easy one to plan. If you enjoy playing pool or ping pong, make room for it. Darts and corn hole out on the lanai is fun. If you play board games or card games, have a designated space for that.

GRACIOUS HOST PROTOCOL

- Always greet guests at the door and make them feel welcome.
- Have a place for guests to deposit purses and belongings.
- If planning to ask guests to remove their shoes before entering your home, let them know before the party. If you are having a large party that includes new acquaintances, colleagues from work, or older people, it is not recommended to have a "no-shoes" policy. Save this one for close friends and family.
- If it is a gift occasion, have a place where gifts can be set.
- Introduce arriving guests to friends already there.
- Give arriving guests directions to the food and drinks.
- After all guests arrive, the host should circulate to make sure everyone has someone to talk to and is enjoying him or herself. Try to steer any conversations away from religion or politics.

- Have someone help keep an eye on the food and drink levels.
- If it is a sit-down event, have place cards at the table (preferred). If not, let your guests know where you would like them to sit. Place the male guest of honor to the right of the host/hostess at the table, and the spouse or date/companion to the right of the host at the table.

The "Silent Signal"
The host/hostess should give a silent signal when to begin the meal by putting your napkin on your lap, and also give the "silent signal" that the meal is over by placing your napkin on the table.

Source: "The Art of the Meal: Simple Etiquette for Simply Everyone" by Patricia Napier-Fitzpatrick

GRACIOUS GUEST PROTOCOL

- Never arrive early for a dinner party but try not to be more than fifteen minutes late.
- Always take a host/hostess gift if you are going to someone's home for a dinner party. Do not take flowers since the host would have to take time from the party to put them in a vase. A potted plant is a better choice. Nor should you take wine that you expect to be opened that evening.
- Do plan to bring a pair of "indoor shoes" with you for the party if you have been walking in the rain or snow. Do take your shoes off before entering the house, if asked to do so, since this is a host's prerogative. (Hopefully, you were forewarned, or should be given slippers to wear in case you've forgotten to bring your "indoor shoes."
- If it is a large party, and your host is not at the door, work your way through the crowd to find the host/hostess and say hello before talking to the other guests.
- Do not hesitate to introduce yourself to others and shake hands with them.
- If you are talking to someone and an unknown person walks up to you both, introduce them, following the rules of proper introductions.
- If you spill something, let the host immediately know and offer to help clean it up.

- If you break something, let the host immediately know and offer to pay for the damage.
- Do not bring another person with you to a party unless you have checked first with the host.
- Do your part to be a gracious and entertaining guest. Make an effort to converse with your dinner companions and other guests at the party.
- Do talk and eat but don't do both at the same time.
- Always thank the host/hostess before you leave, and call or send a thank you note the next day.
- Most importantly, enjoy the party!

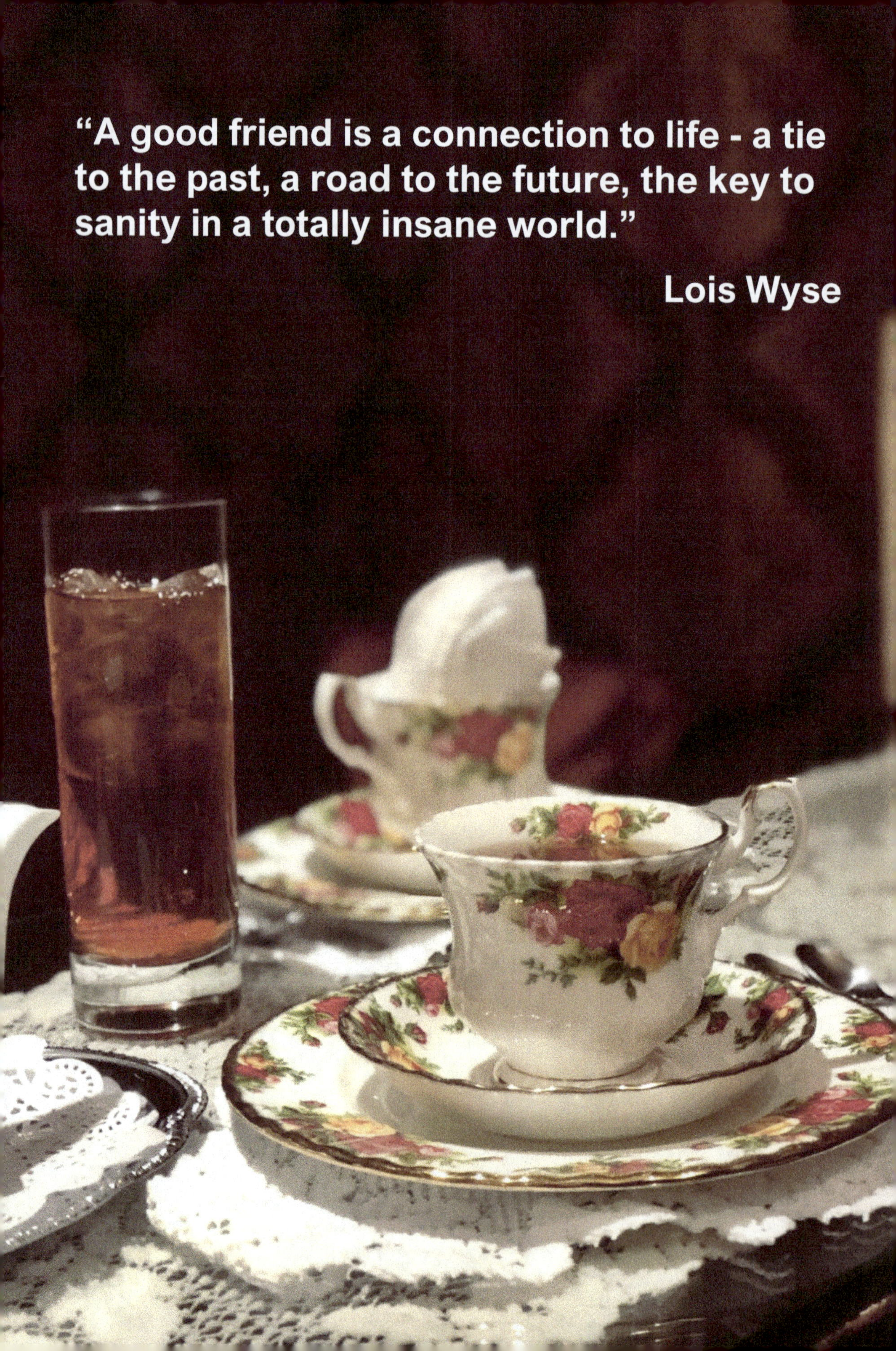

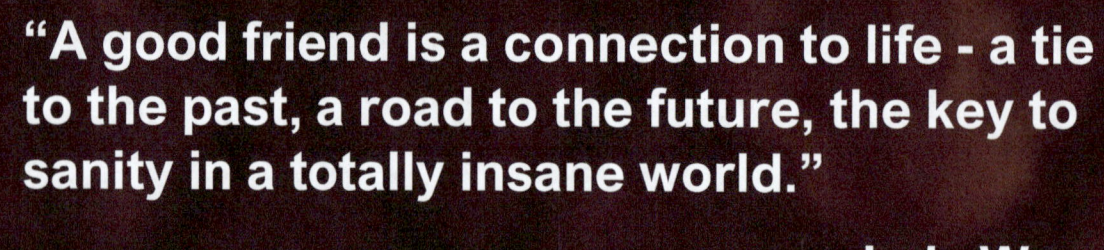

"A good friend is a connection to life - a tie to the past, a road to the future, the key to sanity in a totally insane world."

Lois Wyse

Chapter 3
WEEK ONE
Sending Out the Invitation

Week one is your time for planning and making decisions. Let yourself brainstorm. You want to decide who, what, why, when, and where. Start with a reason to have a celebration! In Appendix I there are lists of creative ideas and options to choose from for having a party that will get you excited. We will develop a 4-week prep timetable for planning your party from start to finish.

The goal of week one is to make all your decisions and arrive at the point of being ready to send out your invitations. This is your starting point and gives you a meaningful direction. It is ideal to send out party invitations three weeks in advance.

However, the holidays are busy, and time is at a premium. If you are part of a large social group with lots of events, the earlier you get that invitation out, the better. You may consider sending out a "save the date" card just to make sure your event is first on everyone's holiday calendar.

Don't worry if you skip details during this early planning period. This is supposed to be fun and stress-free. Remember the ultimate priority is spending quality time with people you care about. Preparation and organization will get you there and is the key to keeping stress at bay.

THEME

This is the easiest place to start developing your concept. Answer the question WHY are you having a party. This will lead to creative ideas and aid in determining the direction of your party.

While a Birthday Party, traditional Thanksgiving Dinner, or Christmas Day Feast may seem easy, there are lots of ways to improve on those traditional holiday celebrations. Plan to do something unexpected. Go the extra mile by creating surprises that will make it memorable.

So, WHY you are having a party? Now begin making decisions on the location of the party, size of the group, menu, time of day, music, then begin making your guest list.

If it's a Party with a Purpose – that's even better!

Perhaps it's someone's birthday. Go all out and make it a big deal! Balloons, cake, candles, the works! Or someone's anniversary? See if you can get hold of some of their wedding pictures. Life is meant to be celebrated!

Holiday Theme Parties

Holiday parties are perhaps the easiest. The house is already decorated, and the spirit of giving is part of the magic. Why not make it a party with a purpose? The holidays are a great time to give back. How about a party where your guests bring a toy that you later deliver to the local fire station? Or some canned goods for the homeless shelter? You can even incorporate your giving into your party planning. Spread the cheer! How about bringing in a local school singing chorale to sing Christmas carols? Perhaps you can reciprocate by contributing to a holiday project at their school.

The theme of your party can dictate everything about your party which makes party planning much easier. You want to create excitement for your guests before they even arrive. Remember, "We're having our annual Christmas party" can be ho-hum. Even an "Ugly Sweater Party," while fun, can be a little overdone. How about **"Come to our Holiday Masquerade Party"** or **"Come to our Mingle and Jingle Christmas Karaoke Party?"** See Appendix 1 for more ideas.

Keep your guest list in mind when choosing your theme but use creativity and start thinking "outside the box" in creating that memorable experience. Keep in mind your traditional Christmas decorations when planning your theme. Setting up a photo booth and taking lots of pictures makes for great memories, especially around the holidays.

Make sure to communicate your plan in your invitation. The Holidays are always a time for giving back. You may want your guests to simply come and enjoy, allowing you to supply everything. Make sure you communicate that as well.

Type of Party
Now that you have found a Reason Why to have your party, it gets easier! The *type* of party often dictates what *kind* of party is best suited for that theme. So, the next decision is to pick what kind of party you want to have: A potluck? A buffet? A dinner party? Once you have chosen your theme, begin to look at the *type* of party you want to have. Be sure to indicate the type of party you are having on your Invitation.

<u>**Potluck**</u> parties are often popular with family and neighbors. The advantage of potlucks is that everyone contributes to the meal:
- Less work for you.
- Less expensive
- You get to taste other people's cooking!

With all that said, I still enjoy furnishing all the food and drinks for my party. It's my gift to my guests. All they need do is show up! I also have more control over the menu, how it is served, and the theme of the party. If you are very confident in your party planning, I would say take total control. However, if you like potlucks and find those advantages important to you, choose a potluck kind of arrangement, but do some micromanaging to keep things on track.

TYPES OF PARTIES

Neighborhood or Family Buffet Potluck
This is probably the most popular type of party, which can be combined with the Driveway Party for a larger crowd. Usually, a Potluck is a party where you supply the space, the plates, napkins, eating utensils, and whatever else the host chooses to contribute. Often the host will also supply the theme, the main course, and the guests bring the supporting dishes, hopefully under the guidance of the host. A center island or a dining room table is a perfect place to set out all the food.

While it may be one of the easiest parties to do, there is an art to it. It's always a good idea to give some kind of direction in what kind of food to bring, and how many people are attending. Ask that they not bring something that needs to be reheated at your house. By giving them some direction, you retain a kind of menu control. For instance, if you are having a Mexican Fiesta party, have an idea about what your guests can bring to develop the theme and menu.

Neighborhood Driveway Party
This is popular for larger groups. Make sure your garage is neat and tidy, at the very least. For my last driveway party, I had a large tent erected inside the garage and put a big rug on the cement floor, hung lights all over, and decorated the tented area like a room; hiding everything that said "garage." We had entertainment and it looked quite festive. People were dancing down the driveway and into the street. It was a crowd of about seventy people. Because of the number of people, I used a combination of the driveway, areas inside the garage and house and used the kitchen counter and lanai for food. I had a bar set up outside the garage.

For this kind of party, keep an eye on the weather since you may need shelter for rain showers in the afternoon. Ask everyone to bring their own chairs, especially if you anticipate a large crowd. It's always handy to have a few of the six-foot long wholesale club tables for large crowds. A couple of large ice chests under the tables work well. Make sure you drape the table to hide the ice chests.

Impromptu

An impromptu party can strike fear into the most experienced party planner! It's important to be ready when everyone decides to stop by your house after an afternoon of golf. Always be prepared. Later in this book, we will develop your go-to list of what you need to have on hand in your pantry and freezer. You will be ready for anything!

Barbecue

If someone in your household is a grill master, put them to work! It's a great way to divide duties. A barbecue is usually casual but can easily be elevated by food choice. Many foods can be grilled beforehand and kept warm in the oven, freeing everyone up to enjoy the party.

Summer kitchens on the lanai are very popular and can be quite elaborate. I have heard of summer kitchens equipped with a full bar, pizza oven, rotisserie, smoker, multiple grills, six-burner stove, wine refrigerator, even television set. That's quite impressive and a great way to entertain.

Traditional Cocktail Party

Offer a full repertoire of tasty appetizers and drinks. Usually, a shorter party is best held about in the afternoon around three or four o'clock and before dinner plans. This can also be a potluck where guests contribute to the menu.

Holiday Open House

A holiday open house allows you to invite more friends than you usually would. If you have a large guest list, stagger the hours to alleviate a traffic jam. Have some guest invitations printed with the hours from one to three o'clock and the other half stating they should come from two to four o'clock. Choose your menu carefully to include those things that can stay tasty over several hours with a minimum of extra preparation.

Traditional Buffet

Plan your menu carefully and do most of your prep work before the party. For control freaks, this is the best choice of party. You have total control over the theme, menu, choice, presentation, and quality of the food.

Traditional Dinner Party
Traditional dinner parties are not as difficult to pull off as you might expect with the proper menu planning. You can bring in additional help to serve. You might also hire a chef from one of the local restaurants to come and cook for you. I have found the best way to keep it manageable is to have a limited number of guests for a more intimate evening. Also, serving the food family-style with large platters of food on the table is a preferred way for food presentation, and one in which you can still enjoy your own party. Plan your menu accordingly.

I once had a five-course Birthday Dinner party for sixteen on my lanai. Admittedly, it was a great deal of work, and I didn't get much of a chance to enjoy my own party. So, while everyone had a wonderful time, this is not something I would recommend without lots of additional help. Everything is learned by experience, please learn from mine.

Large Event Party
A party for twenty people or more need not be intimidating with the right preparation and planning. Use the Master Template in Chapter 5 and multiply the portion recommendations outlined in Chapter 4. Enlist additional help or even hire people. With proper planning, you will have the skills to pull it all together.

DATE

Now that you have decided upon the theme and type of party, ithe t's time to pick a date. The date may be dictated by your choice of theme, such as a Kentucky Derby Day Party or a Super Bowl Party. But if you don't have a specific date indicated, then you need to decide on the date and day of the week.

Giving yourself a month to prepare is a good idea and creates the least amount of stress. Look at the calendar. If you are scheduling a party on the weekend before a holiday (i.e., Halloween, Christmas), you may have some competition with others who are planning parties. Just remember Christmas and Halloween celebrations are the most popular times of the year, so plan ahead!

TIME

The time of day and menu choice are tied together with the theme. For instance, an Easter brunch indicates a time period from about 11 a.m. to 3 p.m. in the afternoon. Make sure you figure in food prep time and clean up time in planning your total time commitment. Your prep time will be dictated by your menu. For instance, if you schedule a party that ends at 9 or 10 p.m. there is little chance of you being in bed by midnight. Similarly, it's not a good idea to schedule a brunch before 11 a.m. unless you like getting up at 4 a.m. to get things set up and ready. **Always include a time the party will end on your invitation.**

GUEST LIST

Make up your guest list early to determine the group you will be hosting. After each name, include a contact number so you can later follow up with your RSVP's. Consider the interests of your guests in your party planning. Is it a karaoke crowd? A "foodie" group? Or a group of "wine lovers"? The success of your party should appeal to the mutual interests of the group you plan to invite. Keep in mind how much seating you will need and how your space will accommodate the number of guests you are planning to invite. The number of guests also will determine your menu and where you hold your party.

WHERE

The theme of your party, the type of party, time of party, and number of guests will help indicate where you can have your party. Are you planning something at home or are you outsourcing? You could choose to have your party at a recreation center, hotel, restaurant, or park.

Having an event at your own home is always more intimate and personal. You can control the music, the food, and the well-being of your guests. You might have a summer kitchen that you would like to use. Eating out on the lanai is wonderful most of the year. Entertaining around the holidays is always fun as you can share your holiday decorations.

Here are some options if you are very popular and have lots of friends:

- The most expensive choice is to rent a room in a restaurant. You can arrange a special menu with the restaurant at a price that you agree on ahead of time; usually a per person rate would apply. You might arrange to have some bottles of wine on the table. Having an open bar can get very pricey. The restaurant choice takes the least amount of work and preparation. You may arrange to bring some of your own decorations if you get a private room. The downside to a restaurant party is that it can be very loud unless you have a private room with a door to close. Other potential downsides are that the service may not be as good as you would like or the food might not be hot as you expected. Their best chef might also be off that night. Perhaps you should ask a few of these questions.
- You can have an Open House at your own house over the course of three to four hours. People will filter in and out. See the Portion Section for adjustments. There are ways to control a large crowd with the invitations by adjusting the printed hours. Some will receive an invitation of hours between 1 p.m. and 3 p.m., and others will receive invitations between 2 p.m. and 4 p.m.
- You can reserve one of the rooms in a local Recreation Center. Check early to reserve and make sure you know all the rules and regulations. Keep in mind that this choice has a high "schlep" factor, a hectic limited timeline, and needs to be planned to the last detail to pull off. ENLIST LOTS OF HELP! Hiring a catering service to bring in the food makes it a little easier, but does remove that personal touch, and does increase the cost substantially.

MENU

Now that you have your theme, type of party, number of guests, and location of your party you can begin to focus on your menu. If you need to order any party platters, meat, or other "helpers," factor that into your plans early on and make sure you order in plenty of time. Also figure in time needed to pick up everything into your final schedule.

In choosing your menu, think in terms of number of items that are hot and cold; what items can be done ahead of time or purchased rather than homemade, and how the food relates to your theme. **Follow the Master Template in Chapter 5 in planning your menu in detail.** It is easiest to plan the main dish first and then plan around that with coordinating flavors and dishes.

Details

Start fleshing out some details. Brainstorm. Is there something that should be communicated to your guests? For instance, is it a masquerade party, or a party where they need to bring something—food, alcohol? Include as many details as possible on the Invitation. Start making your lists. You have more than enough time to fill in all the special details. Try to communicate as much as you can on your Invitation to create anticipation and excitement for your party.

BUDGET

Alcohol is the most expensive component of a party. If your guests bring their own, it is a big saving. Just make sure you have a place where they can make their drinks. Furnish glasses, lemons and limes, mixers, soft drinks, and water. A potluck buffet is the least expensive menu type choice You can always have a great party with a limited budget and some inexpensive creativity. Prioritize your money on food and drinks and you can always get creative in your decorations.

Invitation

Make sure you send out invitations with enough time to get on your guest's calendar during a busy season. Decide HOW you want to invite your guests. To truly elevate the event and make it special, create an invitation and send it to them. Vistaprint.com has a good inexpensive collection that only takes a few days to design, order, and receive. Or you might try Staples for a fast turnaround. Then there is Evite, Shutterfly, minted.com, emails, phone calls, text messages .. . all acceptable, but just not quite as special.

If you are having some trouble getting all the details together, don't worry. Send out a SAVE THE DATE card followed by the invitation, hopefully, within a week. Always ask them to respond back to you with an RSVP. You want to have all the information on the invitation which should include the following Master Invitation Template:

MASTER INVITATION

Theme: (Example: Come to Our Masquerade Party!)
Date:
Time:
Where:
Theme and pertinent corresponding information:
What they should bring:

ALWAYS ask your invited guest to "Répondez s'il vous plaît (RSVP)" by a date about one week prior to the event; earlier if it is a potluck. Include your phone number and contact information. Include a map, if necessary, and as much information as needed.

SUMMARY OF WEEK ONE

This was the first week of an exciting journey where you will bring all of your creativity together in the concept of your party. You have made important decisions that you can now develop to begin your planning. You have gotten to the point that you can share your upcoming event and get your Invitations out to people you want to invite.

During Week One you have made some important decisions:
- Theme
- Type of party
- Date of party
- Number of guests
- Time
- Location of the party

You've decided on your budget, your menu, and the beginning of all the details that will make up what will be a wonderful party and smashing success!

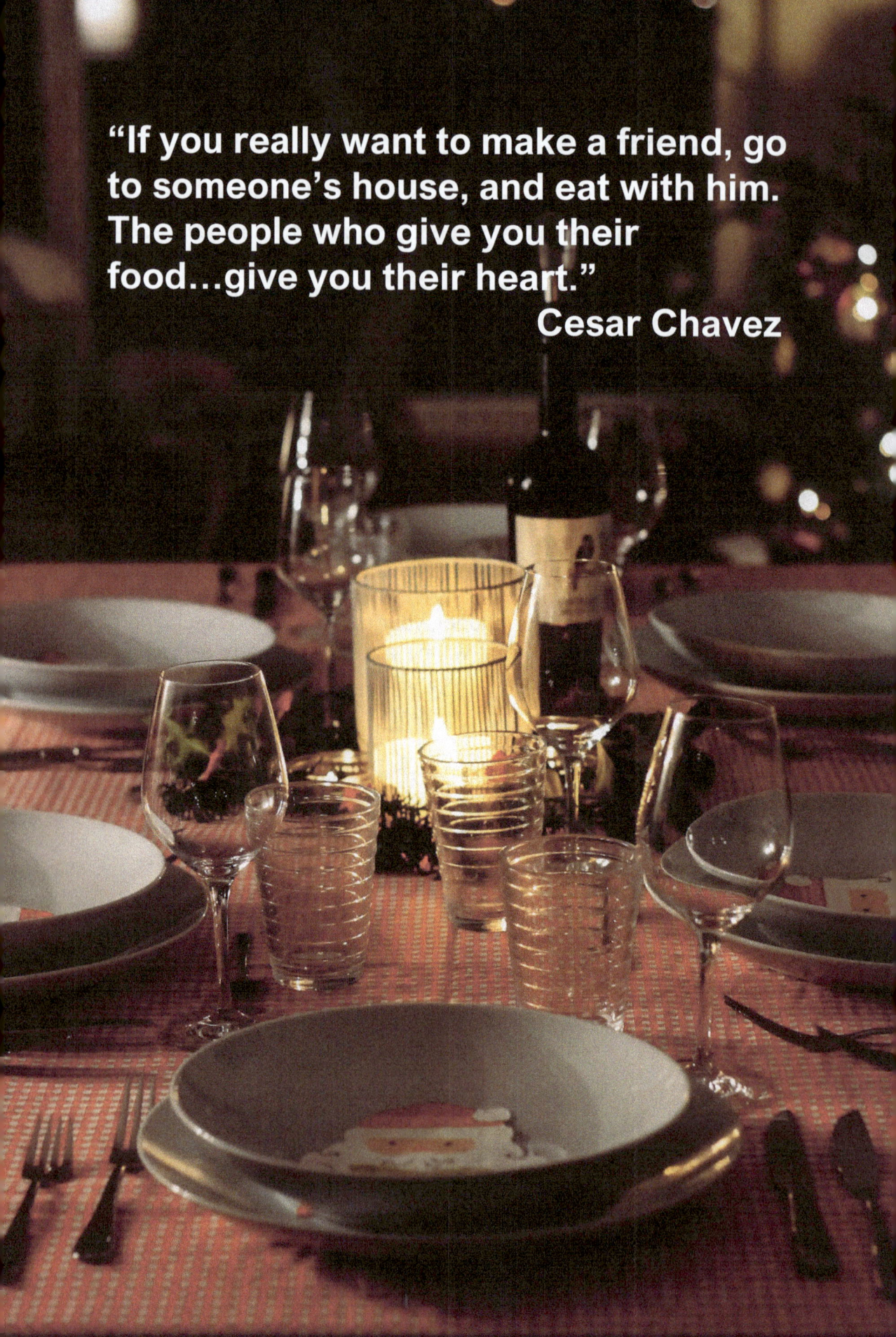

Chapter 4
WEEK TWO
Making Decisions

PART ONE

FINE-TUNING AND DECIDING ON DETAILS

You have decided on your theme, type of party, date, and names of people you are inviting. Now, you have the skeleton of your party and only need to fill in the blanks. Keep making lists and feel free to change something if it's not coming together. There are still some puzzle pieces to work on.

Below are decisions to make in Week Two of your party planning. I hope you are really starting to feel that excitement Let your creativity flow and don't be afraid to think out of the box.

Your Wardrobe
Decide what YOU are going to wear for your party. Have it ready to go, washed and ironed or dry cleaned, so you won't have to worry about it again. There is nothing worse than discovering on the morning of your party that you have nothing suitable to wear. Choose something FABULOUS, comfortable, washable, and preferably not white. Wear something appropriate in colors of your theme and party decorations. Avoid anything too low cut or too short for obvious reasons. Comfortable shoes are an absolute must.

Avoid jewelry that will hang down and get in your way. Keep your hair out of your face. Or you can treat yourself to something new in celebration of all your hard work!

Colors

Decide on the colors of your party. Traditional red and green for the holidays? Plaid? Or maybe gold or silver and white If you are having an Easter brunch, go with pastels, spring flowers, Easter decorations. Start filling in the all-important details. Coordinate the dishes, napkins, tablecloths, and any table runners.

Decorating

Get creative with your party decorating and have it reflect your theme and colors. Having a photo booth or photo corner is always fun. You want you're your guests to say "Wow!" and understand your party theme when they come through the door. Make it special and memorable. Holiday parties are easy since most people decorate homes for the holidays anyway. Christmas decorations can be magical and good for the soul. I encourage you to decorate all you can and enjoy! If you have some limitations in putting up decorations, such as outside lights, see if your budget can handle someone to come and do it for you. These are important touches to set the mood.

Place interior decorations while keeping in mind that you will be having a party. Leave room for additional tables, if needed. Plan ahead and get it done early.

Playlist

Music is very important in setting the tone of your party. It's subliminal but adds so much to the overall experience. Music should be loud enough to hear, but low enough for people to talk. Give some thought to exactly the kind of music you want for your party. This might be a chore for a willing partner. Start early, and make sure it is music you love. Space some of your favorites throughout the playlist to lift your mood and remind yourself to have some fun, too! When compiling your list of songs, think about including Opera for an Italian Dinner or Hawaiian music for a Luau. Perhaps, Frank Sinatra for a New Year's Party.

You might choose to hire outside entertainment for your party. Simply be clear on what you want to achieve. Make sure to book early and confirm with them a week before the event. Best results are usually achieved with someone you have personally seen or heard or who has been recommended to you. Be clear about hours, equipment, wardrobe, costs, and expectations.

Preliminary Shopping
Chapter 5 contains the Master Template to guide you while shopping. It gives you an initial list to take care of this week. You can purchase such items as decorations, alcohol, canned goods, frozen items, paper products, and everything you can buy ahead of time. Also, if there are menu items that can be prepared beforehand and frozen, get those ingredients this week and start things moving. During planning week two, you should have all your party decorations, paper products, napkins, tablecloths, and such in your house by this week's end.

Cleaning up/ Preparation
During Week Two, look at your front door and front yard. Does something need to be cleaned? Any spider webs that can be knocked down around your front door? Would this be a good time to plant some flowers? Do you need a new doormat? Get it done early and out of the way. Set up your lanai if it is part of your plan.

Order Specialty Items
If your party will require any specialty items like table linens, dishes, decorations, and the like, make sure they are ordered early this week. Call and confirm anything you are renting. Now is the time to preorder any meat or party platters.

Extra Help
you will need to hire outside help for set up or serving, contact them this week and go over all the details. Sometimes servers in local restaurants are looking for additional income. Be sure and pay them well.

PANTRY AND REFRIGERATOR BASICS

There are many opportunities to invite people over to your house, perhaps after a golf game or a polo match. It would be wise to decide on a few tried-and-true dishes that you can whip up quickly and effortlessly for those last-minute celebrations.

Following are some sample menus you might try. Once you have decided on which ingredients you need for a few star dishes, make sure to keep these items on hand for just such last-minute entertaining emergencies. Always have a few dishes that are quick and easy to put together and are ready to go. This is an interactive list. Add your favorites!

Pantry Items/ Canned Goods

Chili sauce	Crackers/ sealed
Barbecue sauce	Nuts
Bottle favorite spaghetti sauce	Mints
Black olives	Pickles
Canned mushrooms	Parmesan cheese
Artichoke hearts	Breadsticks
Mayonnaise	Candies

Miscellaneous pasta - penne and mini-penne are good

Freezer

Frozen meatballs - Use in a pasta dish, or with barbecue or chili sauce with toothpicks.

Frozen mini sausages - Sometimes called Little Smokies. Serve with barbecue and chili sauce with toothpicks. Or wrap in pastry dough for old-fashioned pigs in a blanket.

Frozen spinach - There are many appetizers to make and freeze ahead that have spinach as an ingredient. Find a good spinach dip for crackers or bread to have on hand.

Cookie dough - Rolled cookies are delicious and easy to freeze. Multiply and prepare your favorite recipe before baking, then roll the unbaked batch into individual six to eight-inch sections, wrap and freeze with a use-by date and cooking instructions. At the needed time, defrost, slice, and bake.

Refrigerator
Always make sure to have these items on hand before your event. Put them on your shopping list. Use them as a garnish or at the bar. Presentation is everything!

Parsley- Curly is best. Not Italian parsley.
Grapes - green and red —always buy seedless varieties
Cherry tomatoes - Smaller the better.
Lemons
Limes
Carrots,
Radishes
Celery
Sour cream
Assortment of cheeses
Sliced salami or sausages
Lettuce- Try romaine, butter, or curly leaf. Check there are no brown edges.

Wash lettuce in a strainer when it comes home. Separate the leaves and stack on paper towels, then put in zip lock bags still rolled up. When stored like this, lettuce will remain crisper and crunchy for days.

Spice it up
Adding chilis contributes real spice and depth of flavor to your cooking. Become familiar with the different kinds of fresh chilis to add to your favorite recipes. Be aware that chilis have different degrees of heat depending on the time of year. Poblano chilis, for instance, are much hotter in the fall.

Fresh Chilis
Habanero-Incendiary small green or ripened red chilis, about 1-1/2 inches long with a subtle citrus flavor.
Jalapeno-Small, thick-fleshed, fiery chili usually sold green, although red ripened specimens can sometimes be found. Also, can be pickled in brine or smoke fired. The latter are called chipotle chilis and sold dried, canned in vinegar, or in a thick vinegar-based adobo sauce.

Serrano-Small, slim, hot chili found in green or ripened red form, or pickled in brine.
Poblano-The Poblano is a mild chili pepper originating in the state of Puebla, Mexico. Dried, it is called Ancho or Chili Ancho. Stuffed, fresh, and roasted, it is popular in Chiles Relleños Poblanos.

Dried Chilis
Ripe red chilis are commonly preserved by drying. Dried chilis are often soaked in water to soften for easier blending with other ingredients.
Ancho chilis-the dried form of the large, fairly mild fresh poblano, is often used in recipes.

Herbs
Herbs can add a great deal of flavor to your dishes. In Florida, the easiest herbs to grow are basil and mint. They do require attention to watering and some intense sun protection.
Basil-Sweet herb is popular in Italian and French cooking; particularly as a seasoning for tomatoes and tomato sauces. Fresh Basil can be frozen and used later.
Chives-Long, thin, hollow green shoots with a mild flavor reminiscent of the onion, to which it is related.
Cilantro-Green, leafy herb resembling flat-leaf (Italian) parsley, with a sharp, aromatic, somewhat astringent flavor. Also called fresh Coriander or Chinese parsley.
Dill-Fine, feathery leaves with a sweet, aromatic flavor; sold fresh and dried.
Mint-Refreshing herb is available in many varieties, with spearmint the most common. Used fresh to flavor savory and sweet dishes.
Parsley-Popular fresh herb available in two varieties - curly leaf and flat-leaf. The latter, also known as Italian parsley, has a more pronounced flavor and is preferred.
Rosemary-Used fresh or dried, Mediterranean herb with a strong, aromatic flavor well suited to meats, poultry, seafood, and vegetables. Use sparingly except in grilling.
Thyme-Fragrant, clean-tasting, small-leaved herb used fresh or dried as a seasoning for poultry, light meats, seafood, or vegetables.

If using dried herbs, crush them first in the palm of the hand to release their flavor. Or warm them in a frying pan and crush with a mortar and pestle.

Spices

Knowing how to correctly use spices is a great way to make your dishes special and unique.

Allspice-Sweet spice of Caribbean origin with a flavor suggesting a blend of cinnamon, cloves, and nutmeg, hence its name. Sold as whole dried berries or ground.

Cayenne Pepper-Very hot ground red pepper made from dried cayenne and other chilis.

Chili Powder-Commercial spice blend of ground dried chilis and other seasonings such as cumin, oregano, cloves, coriander, pepper, and salt. Purchase in small quantities, as flavor diminishes rapidly after opening.

Cinnamon-Aromatic bark of a type of evergreen tree. Sold whole, dried strips, cinnamon sticks, or ground. Cinnamon sticks are great for stirring in hot chocolate or holiday drinks.

Cloves-Cloves are a rich and aromatic East African spice used to flavor both savory and sweet dishes. Used ground or as whole buds.

Cumin-Middle Eastern spice with a strong, dusky, aromatic flavor. Sold ground or as whole crescent-shaped seeds.

Curry Powder-Generic term for spice blends commonly used to flavor Sound Asian dishes. Among the most common ingredients are cardamom, coriander, cumin, chili, fenugreek, curry leaves, fennel seeds, mace. and turmeric. Purchase in small quantities, as flavor diminishes rapidly after opening.

Paprika-Powdered spice derived from the dried paprika pepper; available in sweet, mild, and hot forms. Hungary and Spain produce the finest paprika. Buy in small quantities ensure a fresh, flavorful supply.

Turmeric-Pungent, earthy-flavored, yellow-orange ground spice that adds vibrant color to any dish.

THE TABLE

Beautiful tablescapes are an art form! Look through magazines for inspiration. HGTV has a new show called "Table Wars" where design skills are tested in creating unique and beautiful tablescapes. Watch it for ideas.

Always have sufficient tables for your guests to sit down and eat. Use your dining room table to express your creativity and bring in your theme. Here you can Introduce party colors through table linens, napkins, dishes, and centerpieces. Make it wonderful and delight your guests.

Candles
The new battery-operated candles are great for safety! Candles on a mirror set a mood and are wonderful as a simple centerpiece. Put one in your guest bath.

Table Runners, Tablecloths, Napkins, Napkin rings
I love table linens! Once in France, I filled my suitcase with wonderful table linens from Provence that I still use to this day. They remind me of that wonderful trip! The colors and quality are amazing and qualify as one of my treasures.

Table runners and napkins are a great way to bring in color and make a statement. Always buy table runners in pairs or even multiples. It's a good way to tie together tables for a larger group, or if you have a small dinner party with only four guests, you can have one runner going north/ south and another going east/west. The runner can also double as a placemat. Get several colors and look to purchase multiples of the ones you like for larger parties. Make sure they are long enough for your table.

A couple of plain white queen flat sheets work for so many things. You can use them to cover the legs of tables, or as an under-cloth for butcher paper. You can put a smaller tablecloth on top, or a runner for a nice look. The white sheet serves as a good base. Of course, you can always use formal tablecloths, but that could mean ironing and proper storage. Again, with formal tablecloths, try and buy multiples.

For most parties you will be using paper napkins. Get two sizes: Dinner-size and cocktail- size. Buy in bulk and invest in quality. It's a great way to bring in color and work with your theme. For a more elevated look, use cloth napkins for the larger napkins. You can buy cloth napkins in bulk (packs of 12) in a good heavy fabric at TJ Maxx. White is always the best choice and can serve double duty to line baskets, or at the bar. Look for the 20x20 size.

Napkin rings are fun and a great decorating tool. You can wrap your plastic eating utensils in a colorful napkin with a coordinating ribbon. Or you can use shells, or beads, or anything that will relate to your theme. Incorporate a name tag in the napkin ring when you are setting the table for a more formal affair.

Centerpieces

This is where you can really make a statement with your theme. However, tall centerpieces do not encourage conversation, and should be removed and replaced before sitting down.

Fresh flowers are always a perfect choice; use this opportunity to reinforce your theme, either in color or style. If entertaining at night, you can incorporate candles into your centerpiece. Give it some thought, make it fun, and make it surprising for your guests. Even if you have a potluck, tables can still be set with table linens and a nice centerpiece.
A thought: keep the centerpieces the same or similar for multiple tables.

Paper Plates

Have two sizes (dinner-size and cake/appetizer-size). Paper dinner plates should be white and heavy (Chinet), and NOT divided. A smaller paper plate can be something reflecting the event and colorful. You will use more of these smaller plates. Buy in bulk.

Chargers

This is a very nice touch for your guests, especially if needing to use a paper plate. They are inexpensive and reusable. Can be plastic or wicker. Buy them by the dozen. A good source is Ross, Dollar Store, or Tuesday Morning. Can also serve double duty as trays.

Silverware

Buy a higher quality plastic in bulk. Michael's the craft store has a good selection of a heavier type. Wrap in napkins with a pretty ribbon before any event, so guests won't have to juggle separate pieces with their plate. Store leftover paper plates, napkins, and silverware in plastic bags between parties.

Plastic Cups
Get two sizes: A clear smaller glass (for wine, mixed drinks), and a larger plastic cup for beer and soft drinks.

Trash Bags
Always have extra bags available and multiple places for people to put their trash.

Take-home Containers
Have foil, plastic bags, and plastic wrap available for both clean up or anything your guests are taking home. One of my favorites are little Chinese takeout boxes ready to go. Buy them on Amazon.

Toothpicks and Skewers
Get an assortment of different lengths. Splurge on some toothpicks with curly colorful ends. I like to have two lengths of bamboo skewers - one about six inches long and the other about ten inches long. *Soak skewers in water beforehand to avoid splinters.*

Formal Parties
Go with your good dishes and silver. If you don't have enough of one set, you can mix and match. You might pick up something lovely at Goodwill. Get creative and make it beautiful!

BAKING, DISHES, PREP

Trays
I like the selection at Ikea and have bought in bulk. I have about five square (13-inch square) black plastic trays, and about ten round silver trays (14-inch round). Both work for food and at the bar.
I also have a couple of glass Christmas trays, too. Buy several of the same kind as it adds a more cohesive look to your presentation.

Baking Sheets
Get four or five and keep them looking good. Never bring out old, stained baking sheets that are nasty in front of guests. Invest in some new ones.

Au Gratin Dishes
I like a 10-inch dish which can work for many uses. It is a great size for dips and cut-up vegetables, bread, or crackers. One benefit is that cooked dips can go right from oven to the table.

Ramekins
Great for sauces and dips. I have many in different sizes. They can go in the oven or microwave for warming things.

Glass Casserole Dishes with Lids
Great for taking things to other parties such as casseroles, brownies, or main dishes.

Plastic Containers with Covers
Have a good selection for prep work and leftovers in all sizes. Plastic shoe-box containers with tops are especially versatile for cookies.

Chafing Dish, Slow Cooker, or Fondue Dishes
A silver chafing dish is very elegant. However, since a chafing dish usually requires Sterno, and has an open flame, it's not one of my favorites since it can be a fire hazard. Also, once the Sterno burns down and depletes, you have to keep watching and replace it. Be sure to buy extra Sterno. Put it on your shopping list
A slow cooker is probably the most versatile. Smaller ones are not that heavy and usually are sufficient. Serving soup in the fall and winter months is one

of my favorite choices for a quick dinner. I have a slow cooker that has three pots allowing me to offer up to three different kinds of soups, which has proven to work very well for a party.

A fondue dish, like the chafing dish, requires Sterno, and you have that open flame situation again. A fondue party has a great deal of charm and offers plenty of nostalgia. It can turn out to be great fun.

Wooden or Marble Cheese Board
Try not to go too big or too heavy.

Baskets
Different sizes always come in handy. You can usually use several of the smaller ones to corral the silverware and napkins, for instance. You will use smaller baskets more than large ones.

Serving Spoons and Tongs
No need for them to match. Just make sure they are clean, in good repair and work for the task on hand.

Insulated Food Carriers
Great for taking your food to potlucks. Have several sizes. If you like to bring something for a potluck that requires a special carrier, like deviled eggs or cupcakes, invest in a good carrier with handle.

Plastic wrap, Foil, Zip Lock Bags, Wax Paper
Get plenty of back-ups and buy in bulk.

Parchment Paper
Trust me! A roll of parchment paper is invaluable and used for so many things. Lining the baking sheet keeps it clean and minimizes clean-up.

Doilies
An absolute yes. Nothing will elevate your presentation more than doilies under your food. Get several sizes - round, oval, and rectangle. They absorb juices from your food and give a professional look to your presentation.

Cupcake holders and Small Paper Holders
These are great for individual bites and a variety of other uses. Buy a variety of them.

Butcher Paper
I always have a roll of butcher paper on-hand. It's useful for so many things! A roll will cost about $15 at Sam's Wholesale Club or Ikea and will last a very long time. One of my very favorite things is to spread out butcher paper over a tablecloth just like it's done in a fancy restaurant. Or even spread it over a bare table. Then, put out a glass of crayons and encourage everyone to write a message about the party and sign it. You'll enjoy their messages while you clean up! Butcher paper is a great table covering for a crab and lobster-boil or shrimp party. All the shells just stay on the paper and are easily cleaned up.

Tissue Paper, Assortment of Ribbon
Ribbon is a great decorating material. It adds color and joy to the room. I purchase higher end grosgrain ribbon in several widths and colors. Wired ribbon works well too. Both are great for tying in your color scheme, tying up your silverware, or any number of uses. Tissue paper is useful for gift bags or containers for your guests. Buy a big supply at Christmas closeouts to last all year.

Lighting
Miniature and small white lights always lend a special kind of magic at a night event. Try putting them in clear vases, or string them in nearby trees, on top of cabinets, or strung on the lanai for any season. The lights are magical. I have clear Command Hooks attached to my screened birdcage to support miniature lights for a great look. But I don't suggest leaving string lights outside year-round because of rain and occasionally strong winds. However, with hooks already in place, it's a snap to string lights and plug them in whenever it looks like a party!

THE TRAVELING FEAST

If you are invited to bring a dish to a potluck, make sure you have a safe way to get your delicious dish there. If you take a hot dish, don't bring it over cold expecting the hosts to heat it. Take it already hot in an insulated carrier.

Have go-to items you like to bring? Invest in the best carrier. For instance, one thing I like to bring is cupcakes. Another is deviled eggs. I invested in special carriers for just those purposes which makes certain they arrive in great shape. Don't forget to bring your own serving utensils, too.

Invest in some Styrofoam coolers for taking anything that needs to stay cold. They don't have to be expensive or very large. Have several cold gel packs in the freezer to help keep your foods cold until you arrive at your destination.

PLANNING PORTIONS

When you're having a party, you'll need to determine the right amount of food to serve. You want your guests to have enough to eat so they feel satisfied, but you don't want a ton of leftovers either.

Many factors come into play when planning the amount of food to provide including length of party, type of food, composition of men and women, and richness of food you plan to serve. The time of day or night is also important. An afternoon cocktail party requires much less food than a dinner barbecue. Not all gatherings feed equally, nor should you feel pressured to overfeed the gathering. It isn't necessary. Each time you make a recipe, you will get a better gauge on the size of portions to serve.

Portion Size per Person
Once you start getting a rough idea of the number of guests, you can start putting together your shopping list.

Portions/ Appetizers and Cocktail Parties
- When hors d'oeuvres are the meal, plan on <u>four to eight bites per person per hour</u>.
- For longer parties and larger guest lists, increase the number of selections offered.

- If a meal is included, cut back to <u>three or four appetizers per person per hour</u>.
- For fresh fruit, plan on <u>one-half cup per person</u> to do the job. With veggies, estimate about <u>eight to ten pieces per person</u>. Have plenty of dip available as well.

Portions/ Full Meals
- If offering a choice of dishes, try to anticipate which will be most popular and have extras on hand. Serving sizes will depend on type of entree, so if you serve a buffet, make sure you have enough for everyone to sample each dish. Side dishes can be tricky, but you can estimate about <u>four ounces of each dish as a serving</u>.
- For potato, pasta, or other prepared salads, one gallon will feed 20-25 people.
- For leafy vegetable salads, plan on about <u>one cup per person, before dressing</u>. Always buy an extra bottle of dressing.
- Poultry, Meat or Fish – plan on <u>six ounces per person</u> when you have one main dish, <u>eight ounces when you offer two or more main courses.</u>
- Rice or Grains – Plan 1-1/2 ounces as a side dish, two ounces in a main dish such as risotto.
- Potatoes - five ounces per person
- Vegetables - four ounces per person
- Beans - two ounces per person as a side dish
- Pasta - two ounces for a side dish, three ounces for a first course, four ounces for a main dish.
- Green Salad - one ounce per person undressed weight.

Portions/ Desserts

It's best to offer desserts as single servings. You can easily calculate how many you will need. Have extras on hand for big eaters or those with a particularly sweet tooth.
- One 9" layer cake will serve 10-12 people; one 9" pie will serve six to eight people.
- At the end of a three-hour dinner party, your guests are not going to want a big slab of cake or wedge of pie. Just a little something sweet will suffice. A flourless chocolate cake

recipe might be nice as it feeds eight, but you can slice in into 12 slivers and garnish each with a dollop of fresh whipped cream and raspberries to fill out the plate. The goal is to leave your guests wanting more, not waddling home uncomfortably stuffed.

- You can always do a creamy dessert such as a pudding or mousse.
- A scoop of flavorful ice cream, sherbet, or gelato works well - figure five ounces per person.
- There is always the European tradition of fruit and cheese after a meal.
- Small bowls of mints or chocolates on the table is a nice finish.
- Parties where desserts are the main feature requires a larger selection and many more servings. Be generous.

General Tips and Guidelines

The most important factor is the number of guests. That determines the amount of food you will need, but there are a few other considerations, too. Once you decide on the number of guests to invite (always include yourself,) you won't have a firm count of attendees until you count all RSVP's. So, unless you are having a potluck, begin calling your guests one week after issuing the invitation to begin getting an idea on how to plan the menu. Make sure you ask guests to RSVP, but if you don't hear from someone, it's safest to assume he or she WILL attend.

- Open houses allow you to invite more people but expect them to only stay part of the time. You can consider cutting portions in half.
- The time of day dictates the types of food you will serve. If the party is scheduled at mealtime, for example, you'll be expected to serve something substantial. If your party is at night or mid-afternoon, you can simply serve desserts, appetizers, or snacks.
- Always round UP your estimates, don't round them down.
- Anticipate which food selections will be most popular and serve more of them than general portions guidelines suggest. For example, shellfish appetizers are always popular, so serve as much as your budget allows.

- The more choices you offer, the smaller your calculation of individual portion size can be.
- Assume your guests will taste everything at a buffet, but tastings will be small. However, overall consumption per individual will be GREATER than with fewer choices.
- Add bulk items to your menu. For a sit-down dinner have plenty of bread or rolls to satisfy any big eater. When hosting a cocktail party, nuts, olives, pretzels, etc., provide a little extra security that you'll have enough for all, and they require no extra work.
- Don't repeat the main ingredient. For example, don't serve a shrimp appetizer and have shrimp as the main dish.
- Consider colors of the food to be served together. Make sure there is colorful variety.
- Offer both hot and cold foods on a buffet.
- Mix textures and varieties such as a crisp potato galette served with a soft vegetable puree as side dishes.

Coming up in Week Two – Part Two "Setting the Bar.

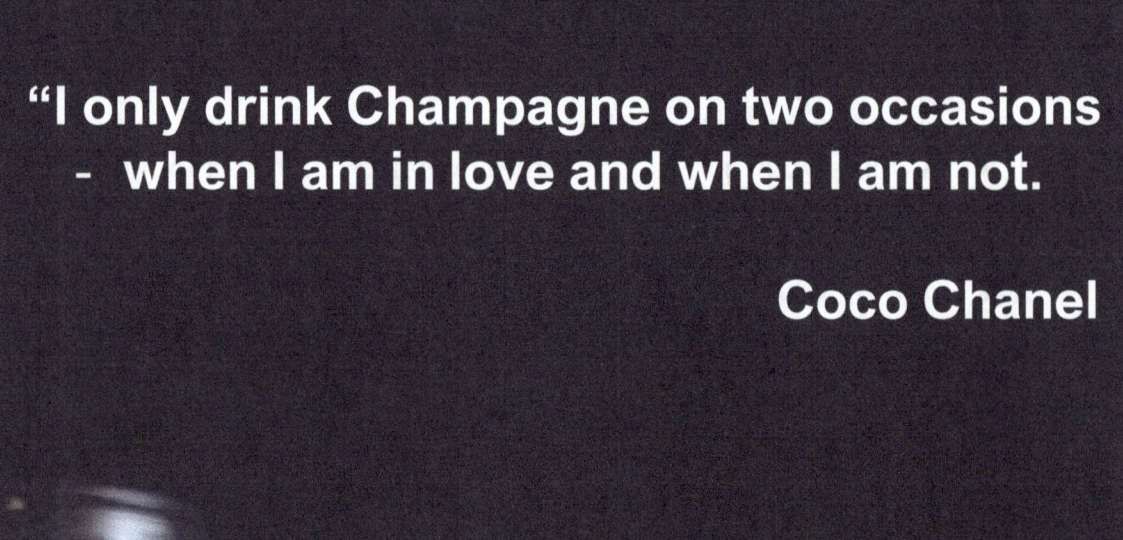

"I only drink Champagne on two occasions - when I am in love and when I am not.

Coco Chanel

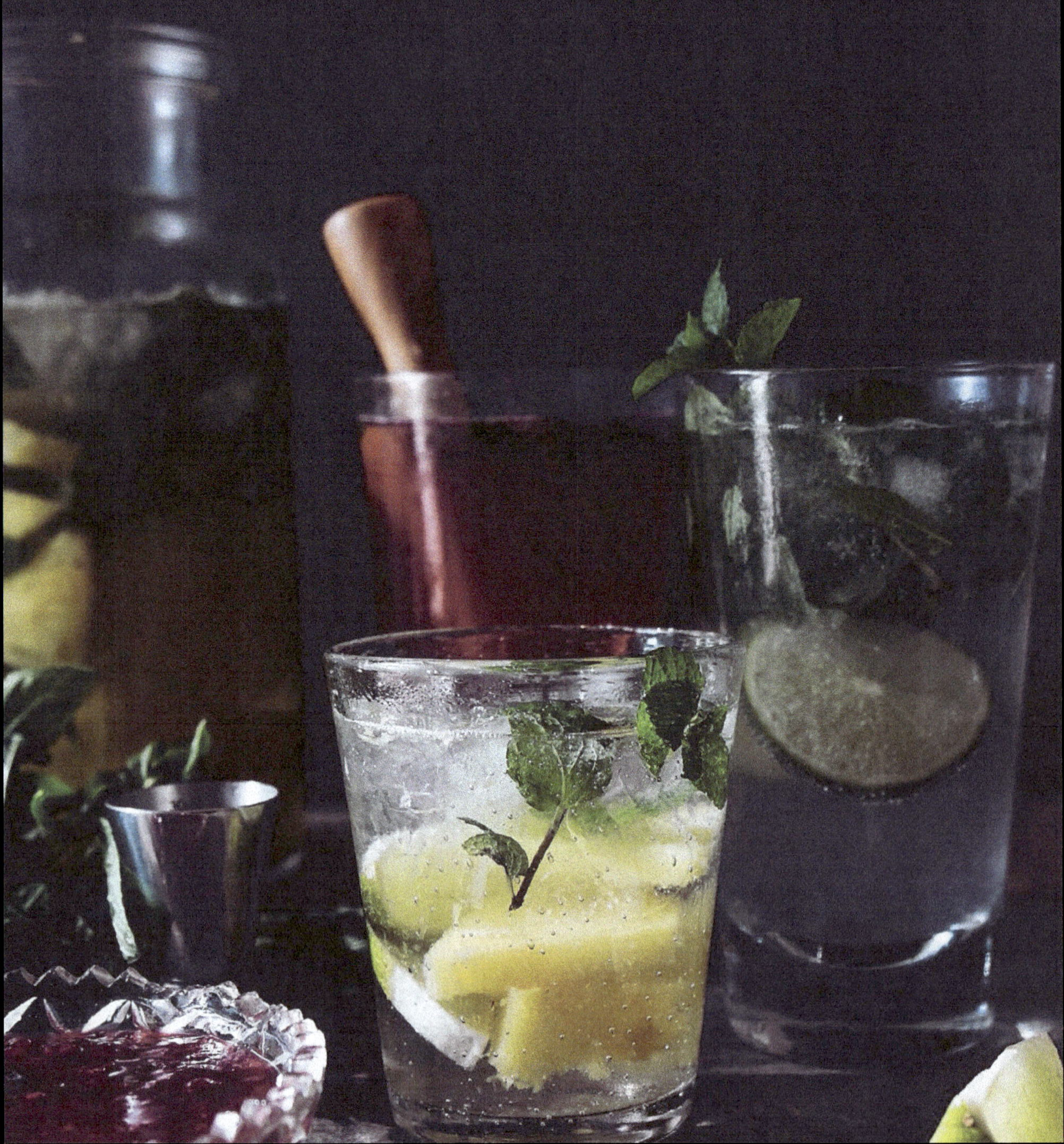

Chapter 4
WEEK TWO
Setting the Bar

PART TWO

Below is a guide for your ultimate Basic Bar Set Up. Much of this is governed by how often you entertain, what your spirit preferences are, and how much you want to invest. Many times, it's popular to have parties where everyone brings their own choice of alcohol. Since alcohol is the most expensive component in entertaining, that plan allows people to entertain more often while guests are sure to have drinks they prefer. Even if you choose to ask guests to bring their own liquor, have a minimal bar set up and ready for your guests.

Remember to have a policy for ways to deal with a guest who has imbibed too much to make it home safely. Deciding ahead of time how you will handle such a situation is the best way to prepare for anything that could become awkward.

BRING YOUR OWN BOTTLE (BYOB) PARTY

You should have the basic barware: Ice, water, non-alcoholic mixers, and condiments on hand and set up. Basic condiments include lemons, limes, cherries, and olives. It's also nice to have a few bottles of wine setting out along with some popular beer, soft drinks, and water.

Another idea is to have a non-alcoholic version of your signature punch that is compatible with your theme and to which a chosen alcohol can be added. This will appeal to both your drinkers and non-drinkers.

WHERE TO PLACE THE BAR

A bar can be anything from a liquor cabinet, small chest, tiki bar, or bar cart. You might utilize a closet, or even use the laundry room in your home for a portable bar set up. The main thing to remember is that it should be placed AWAY from the food and easily accessible to your guests without causing a traffic jam.

It's a nice touch to have a bowl of nuts, pretzels, and maybe mints near the bar which can be a permanent set-up or one you make up just for your parties.

I have a desk in my living room that I use every day. When entertaining, I clear it off and move it against the wall in the living room to use as a bar. It works perfectly for me. I have seen extravagant liquor cabinets and portable bars also used. Do what makes you happy and works for you.

STORAGE

Alcohol should be stored in a cool, dry place away from sunlight. Vermouth should be stored in the refrigerator. Vodka, tequila, white wine, champagne, and Bailey's Irish Cream are often stored in the refrigerator as well. The more a bottle is depleted, the faster it should be drunk, as the amount of air in the bottle will determine its quality. Always make sure the top is on tight.

BARWARE

Tools of the Trade
Stock your bar with the following items:

- Bar Spoon – long and usually stainless steel
- Toothpicks - standing in a small container
- Muddler (for mojitos)- kind of like a little club
- Blender (optional)
- Jigger (shot glass)- Have several on hand
- Cocktail shaker- stainless steel is best
- Strainer (usually comes with a shaker)
- Keurig coffee maker (for coffee drinks)
- Straws, stir sticks
- Little umbrellas
- Can Opener
- Wine Opener
- Bar towels/ White large napkins
- Cocktail Napkins

Ice
Ice is very important to have on hand and doesn't need to cost a lot or require buying large bags beforehand. Several days before an event, begin emptying your Freezer ice maker into heavy zip lock bags and stocking up. This is the ideal size to empty directly into your ice buckets. Here's what you'll need

- An ice bucket (or use a large bowl) for the bar
- Tongs to use while putting ice into drinks.
- An additional ice bucket for keeping soda, beer, white wine, and champagne cold at the bar.
- A larger container (ice chest) kept in the garage or under the bar with backups of more cold items. Make this a little more attractive by using a galvanized bucket or camouflaging it. Use the colors of your party.
- Put wine and beer in an ice bath (ice and water) with some salt one-half hour before guests arrive.

Glassware

- Glasses – Have 6 to 8 each of three types: short, tall, and stem - Clear glass, heavy, no ornamentation
- Stemmed wine glasses – Have 8-12 available
- Have 2 to 3 pitchers for water, juice, and other non-alcoholic beverages
- Have 6 to 8 champagne flutes (optional)
- Have 6 to 8 martini glasses (optional)

STOCKING THE BAR

Basic Liquors

- Cognac - for Sidecars, Brandy Milk punches, Crusts, Daisies, and Smashes
- White rum - for daiquiris and mojitos
- Dark rum - good for many kinds of parties
- Gin - for Martinis, Gin and Tonics, Tom Collins
- Bourbon - for Manhattans, Old Fashions, Whiskey Sours
- Vodka - for Vodka Tonics, Screwdrivers, Vodka Martinis, Vodka Collins, Bloody Marys
- Tequila - for Margaritas, Sunrises, Palomas. Best to stick with 100% Agave Tequila
- Scotch - always a favorite

While you may have your personal favorites, I suggest investing in several name brands for your basic bar.

Optional Liquors

- Sherry
- Kahlua
- Flavored vodkas
- Cognac
- Brandy

Specialty after-dinner drinks are nice to have such as Baileys, Peppermint Schnapps, special brandies, and more.

Mixers
- Cointreau - Natural orange flavor, not too sweet
- Red Vermouth - For Manhattans
- White Vermouth - For Martinis
- Bitters - It is not what the name suggests, but it helps other flavors blend well.
- Simple Syrup

Miscellaneous
Have a variety of the following items on hand especially individual bottles of water and soft drinks.

- Water, Club Soda, Tonic, Coke, Collins 7 up, Ginger Ale, Worcestershire sauce, Tabasco Sauce.
- Orange Juice, Tomato Juice, Cranberry Juice, Pineapple Juice (optional), Grapefruit Juice (optional)
- Condiments
- Green olives, Lemons, Limes, maraschino cherries, cocktail onions; mint for mojitos
- Salt, Pepper, celery salt, sugar
- For Bloody Mary's- celery stalks, shrimp, olives, cocktail onions

Non-Alcoholic Drinks
Always have the usual drinks available for non-alcoholic drinkers such as water, coke, tonic, ginger ale, and juice. I really like the idea of a signature non-alcoholic punch that is just a little special, mirrors the theme, and is thoughtful because it includes everyone.

Beer, Wine, and Sparkling Wines
Stock a few of the most popular beers and include a "light" beer choice. Always provide a tall beer glass (either plastic or glass.)

Have a few wines open and available when your guests arrive. Red wine might include a Merlot and perhaps a Pinot Noir and can be at room temperature. White wines such as Pinot Grigio and Chardonnay are popular and should be served chilled. Rosé wines have become popular and are a light alternative to be served chilled.

As an optimistic person, I think every refrigerator should have a bottle of champagne, always cold and ready for life's unexpected celebrations. Obviously, if you have a party where champagne would complement your theme, have several bottles available. Champagne is also a popular mixer for different kinds of punch, or Mimosas for brunch.
Another popular sparkling wine is Prosecco, which is also versatile.
Not as sweet as champagne, still, Prosecco is celebratory and very tasty.

When purchasing sparkling wine, don't purchase the least or most expensive brands. Find a good mid-price sparkling wine that you like.

General Guidelines for Alcohol

- It is always better to have too much than too little.
- Don't forget the ice at one pound per guest
- For a two-hour party, plan on three glasses, three drinks, three napkins per person.
- Add one drink for every hour thereafter

WINE BASICS

This can be overwhelming. The aisles of wine and many different labels and blends can be so confusing! Below are some wine basics that can help you navigate what you need.

Learning about wines begins with knowing types of grapes. The most important ones are the Big Six, sometimes known as the "power elite." These grapes are the foundation for some of the world's best wines and are grown throughout the world. Climate, soil, and winemaking techniques differentiate the wines produced from them.

WHITE WINES

Chardonnay
The most popular white wine, by far, and top-selling varietal is chardonnay as the first choice for many wine drinkers. As soon as you pour a glass, you'll notice the yellow gold color and rich aroma. It tends to be full bodied with a creamy or buttery texture. Spice, vanilla, toast, and oak flavors are often found in chardonnays that have been aged in oak barrels.

Sauvignon Blanc
Sauvignon Blanc wines are refreshing and light. This varietal usually has strong aromas of citrus (grapefruit, lemon, and lime) and are almost always dry. France's Sancerre wines are also made from this grape variety, and they can have more herbaceous or "earthy" notes like cut grass or green bell peppers. It pairs well with many dishes, especially seafood and vegetarian menus.

Riesling
This grape produces wines that range from very dry to very sweet and usually has the lightest body of the noble white wine grapes. The bottle's back label may have the International Riesling Foundation's scale indicating its level of sweetness. Growing regions also are clues to the style and taste. German Rieslings tend to be sweet and light bodied; Austria and France's Alsace Region offer the cleanest flavors and are among the most food-friendly wines. A good Riesling is well-balanced with its sweetness offset by high levels of acidity.

RED WINES

Pinot Noir

Wines made from pinot noir grapes are lighter, both in color and body. They are also food friendly, especially with a classic pairing of grilled salmon or a savory chicken dish. Generally grown in cool climates, these grapes can be temperamental and difficult to grow; hence prices tend to be higher. Cranberry and red cherry flavors are found in wines produced in cooler climates (Oregon, Burgundy,) while wines from moderate zones (California) exhibit flavors of raspberries and black cherries. Pinot noir is also a grape used for French Burgundy wines.

Merlot

Merlot wines lost favor with oenophiles in the early 2000's because vintners overplanted vines in response to the popularity of the "merlot mantra" of the 1990's and often used the wrong kind of soil and climate. Consequently, the wines were not good. Then came the 2004 movie "Sideways" which really disparaged the varietal. Luckily, winemakers are winning fans back with medium-bodied merlots that have the tannins, acidity, and flavors to make them excellent choices with or without food. The silky, round texture makes them more appealing to some people than tannic cabernets.

Cabernet Sauvignon

Cabernet Sauvignon is the top selling red varietal because of its intensity and full-body flavors. The vines grow well all over the world, and the hardy grapes allow winemakers to achieve consistency and good taste. An excellent cabernet can be found at any price point, whether you are on a tight budget or can afford to splurge. And when it comes to pairing with a steak dinner, it's a classic choice.

Sorting it all out

Wines are often described as light, medium, or full-bodied in referencing their "tasting notes." The best way to understand the concept of "body" is to think about the texture of milk. Equate skim milk with pinot noir and Riesling; whole milk has medium body, like merlot and Sauvignon Blanc. Finally, there is rich, heavy cream, which coats your tongue. This is what chardonnay does with its oaky or buttery flavors. Cabernet Sauvignon is often considered the crème de la creme of wines because of its full body richness and intense flavors.

A great way to taste the difference among these varietals is to sample them side-by-side. Have a light cheese and some bread or wine crackers so you can see how food changes the flavors. Serve white wines and the pinot noirs slightly chilled, but not too cold because that will mask the flavors.

TIPS FOR PAIRING WINE AND FOOD

To create a great food and wine pairing means finding a balance between the components of a dish and the characteristics of the wine.

- The wine should be more acidic than the food.
- The wine should be sweeter than the food.
- The wine should have the same flavor intensity as the food.
- Red wines pair best with bold flavored meats (e.g., red meat)
- White wines pair best with light-intensity meats (e.g., fish or chicken)
- It is better to match the wine with the sauce than with the meat.

A "contrasting pairing" creates balance by contrasting tastes and flavors. More often than not, white wines, sparkling, and Rosé wines create contrasting pairings.

A "congruent pairing" creates balance by amplifying shared flavor compounds. Red wines will most likely create congruent pairings.

Signature Punch

In the 17th Century, employees of the British East India Company discovered punch, a beguiling combination of spirits, water, lemon, sugar, and spices that became synonymous with good cheer and festive celebrations all over Europe.

I encourage you to have a Signature Punch in your arsenal; something special that you love and can easily be put together. Having a punch available is an inexpensive way to serve alcohol (or not) and can be a great addition to the theme of your party.

When making the punch, you can add alcohol to your recipe, or offer it non-alcoholic, with complimentary alcohol nearby for guests to add to their liking. If you are making a punch with alcohol, keep it light. Your guests don't want to have a hangover the next day. Make sure your punch is displayed in a punch bowl with an easy scoop or ladle, with glasses nearby. Freezing fruit in ice cubes is a good way to get texture and color.

There are literally dozens of punch recipes online. A common term for a punch is a Sangria, which can be a real winner in this category. A Sangria can be made with wine, vodka, rum, brandy, or any number or combination of other liquors.

According to the Food Network:

"Sangria is the mixture of wine, fruit, sweetener, and sometimes liquor and is capable of bringing such happiness that science should consider it an antidepressant."

The key to getting it to that sparkling state is to add club soda or champagne right before serving.

Always try whatever you are serving before offering it to your guests. Appendix 1 has some recipes that will work for most parties. Some even sound wonderful for a summer afternoon!

SUMMARY OF WEEK TWO

This has been a busy week with many decisions and the development of your party. By now, you should have decided upon your:

- Wardrobe
- Colors
- Decorating
- Playlist
- Preliminary shopping needs
- Paper products
- Ordered specialty items
- Reviewed supplies and tools
- Decided on tables
- Decided on portions
- Liquor and alcohol
- Signature punch
- Wine and wine pairings

This is shaping up to be quite a party!

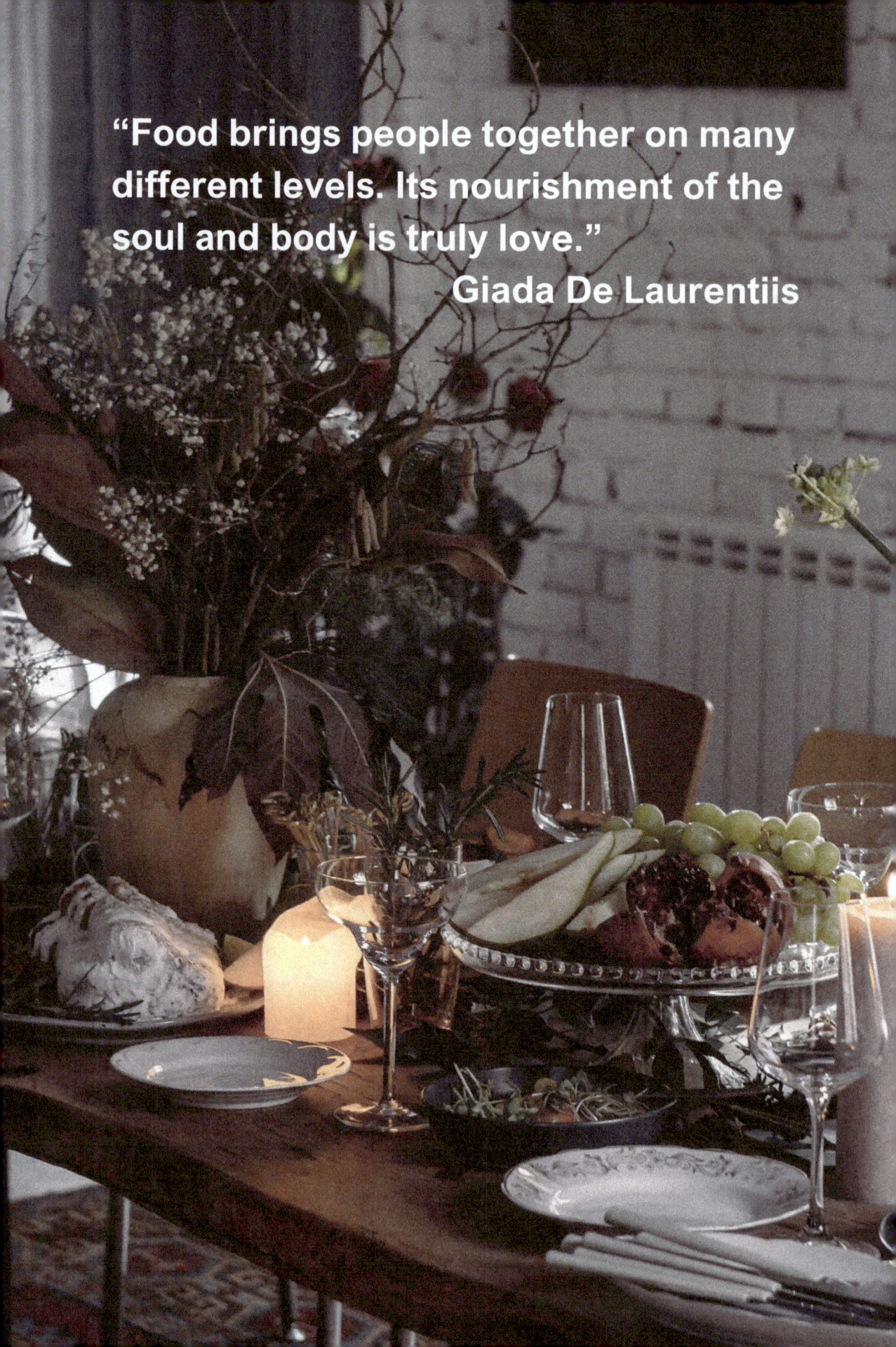

"Food brings people together on many different levels. Its nourishment of the soul and body is truly love."
Giada De Laurentiis

Chapter 5
WEEK THREE
Getting It Under Control

PART ONE

FINAL DETAILS

This is the week when you get a handle on stress. This is the week when your plan comes together, and you gain control. This is when you organize and do everything possible ahead of time, then cross it off your list.

Hostess Gifts
It's always a nice touch to send something home with your guests. Give some thought as to which item, how to wrap it, and what you need to assemble your take-home gifts.

After a Christmas party, I once sent home a little loaf of banana bread with fancy coffee for the next morning. After an Easter Brunch, I sent home some wonderful chocolates. Or if you can find something that will enhance the memory of your party, even better. You might send home a photo of the evening in a small picture frame if you have a Polaroid camera or you can print from your iPhone. Get creative; it needn't be expensive; just thoughtful.

Detail Planning

Start doing some in-depth planning. What are you serving? What ingredients do you need? How much prep work will it entail? What pots do you need to cook? Can you make it ahead of time? Which dishes will be used to serve? **This week you will be using a master template located later in Chapter 5 Part 2.** Write everything down. Make your lists. That is how everything will start coming together beautifully!

Inventory

During this week, make sure you have enough trays, serving dishes, and cookware. If you are short on something, borrow from a neighbor or friend, or run to the store and pick it up.

Inventory will include food you have on hand, and what is already in your freezer, pantry, and refrigerator. It's amazing how we forget what's already on hand, or at the back of a pantry shelf. Check expiration dates! You may have a can of something you need for your party that will save a little money. In the words of Martha Stewart: "That's always a good thing!"

Bar

Begin stocking your bar. Hopefully by now, you've decided on where you are going to place your bar, how it will flow for your guests, and what supplies you'll need. Also, hopefully you have decided if you would like to have a Signature Punch for your party. Make a separate list including any paper products, stir sticks, straws. Will you be needing lemons, limes, cherries, or other fruit? Those need to go on the Master Shopping List If you are having a Signature Punch, make sure to add those ingredients to the Master Shopping List, as well. Planning on some beautiful frozen floating berries in your punch? Remember those as well! Every component part needs to be counted or added to your shopping list.

Decorations

This is a fun part, and hopefully, it will wake up your playful side - enjoy it! Decorating to the music on your party playlist should help get you in the mood. Begin putting together decorations for the party. Put together your centerpieces, check your table linens. Put up any lights. This will help you put the mental picture together. Decorations are an opportunity to introduce the unexpected or playful aspects of your event. Decorate with a smile and the smiles will come back to you!

Invitations
Continue following up on the reservations. It's easy to do with your guest list, the menu, and a glass of wine in front of you! One reason I like mailed invitations is that it reminds people to acknowledge your invitation. Getting to a final number is really important to you as the host. It influences your menu choices, portions, and supplies.

So, get on the phone or start texting your guests with a reminder of the event; ask if they will be coming? If it's a potluck, this is a great opportunity to find out what they are bringing, and to offer any guidance, if necessary. For instance, maybe someone else is already bringing a similar dish. Try to have an alternative suggestion ready in that case along with what would work with your menu and plan. Or some people will say "yes, they want to come .. " but have no idea what to bring. That's when you fill in the blanks and advise them from your master menu. Try and be enthusiastic with your contacts and try to give them a glimpse of what you are planning which will add to their anticipation.

Scheduling
Schedule any housecleaners, landscapers, or other staff. If you are hiring help, confirm the date and time with them.

Ice
Start bagging ice from your refrigerator. This has become a joke in my classes. I absolutely HATE buying bags of ice! They are heavy, and sometimes partially melt or leak on the way home. Besides, I get ice for free from my refrigerator! I know…not a big deal, right? But I have found an advantage in bagging my own ice in manageable zip lock bags. It's usually just the right amount I need, and lots easier than handling that big bag of ice from the grocery store. Another advantage is that you won't have to deal with a leftover ice mess, because it is rare that you will go through a large bag of ice for most events.

Lighting

Evaluate your lighting sources. What kind of mood are you shooting for? If it's a potluck, make sure people can see the food. Formal dinner party with soft jazz playing? Keep the lighting low. Battery-operated candles are a godsend, both in safety, cost, and longevity. Stock up on them and batteries, too! You might invest in some solar lighting for your front walkway. It's always a welcoming addition for your guests and enhances the front of your house.

Initial Shopping Trip

After finalizing your menu from the Master Template in Chapter 5 – Part 2 you will have your Initial Shopping List. Purchase as many items as you can during this week and lighten the load of things to do during your final week.

Pulling it all together

Begin doing EVERYTHING you can ahead of time. Put the napkins and silverware together and tie them with a ribbon for a buffet while you're watching television. Can you put together your centerpieces? Do it! Make sure any table linens are pressed and ready to go.

Sample Menus

Here are sample menus that you may inspire you. These are submitted just to get your creative juices going, perhaps, help you formulate some "go to" menus of your own. List them and keep them in your binder.

Impromptu/ Bare Basics
Keep it easy and make sure it is something you can put together in a hurry.
- Nuts
- Pretzels
- Mini hot dogs (from the freezer) heated in barbecue sauce
- Grapes
- Cheese and salami or sausage

Easy Cocktail Party Menu
Hot:
- Meatballs (freezer) in bottled chili sauce (stovetop)
- Hot artichoke dip and sliced French bread or crackers (assemble day before, heat in oven)
- Stuffed mushrooms (assemble day before and heat in oven)

Cold:
- Ham roll-ups (assemble day before)
- Salami and cheese tray (assemble day before)
- Veggie tray with Hidden Valley Ranch Dressing or hummus (prepare day before)
- Deviled eggs (assemble day before)

Shopping List: Frozen meatballs, bottled chili sauce, parmesan cheese, canned artichoke hearts, mayonnaise, crackers, mushrooms, stuffing mix, eggs, sliced ham, canned asparagus, cream cheese, salami, 2-3 kinds of sliced cheese, carrots, cherry tomatoes, parsley, celery, sliced peppers

Supplies needed: 5 trays, 1 large ramekin, slow cooker

Easy Brunch Menu
Hot:
>Bacon (cook ahead and warm in oven)
>Sausage (brown ahead and warm in oven)
>Ham (optional; warm in oven)
>Potatoes (prepare ahead and warm in oven)
>French Toast casserole (assemble ahead and warm in oven)
>Eggs- Only thing that needs to be done last

Cold:
>Fruit Salad
>Various muffins, scones, croissants/ butter and jam
>Supplement with Bloody Marys (don't forget the celery!) and/or mimosas

Warm Casual Dinners

Soup and Salad:
A large tureen of soup (or several choices) with at least three kinds of salads. A pasta salad, green or Caesar salad, and potato salad

Grilled Cheese and Soup:
Make the sandwiches and brown on stove before guests arrive. Let cool and cut off crusts and put on cookie sheet and keep warm in oven. Try different kinds of cheeses. Pair with the old favorite tomato soup or a choice of soups that can be made ahead.

Mexican Buffet
Beans, warm tortillas, browned beef, and chicken made ahead of time, sliced lettuce, tomatoes, salsa, sour cream, rice, tortilla chips. Let guests assemble their own! Supplement with margaritas.

More formal Buffet
Spiral sliced ham - don't forget mustard and horseradish sauce
Lasagna -make ahead and put in oven. Makes house smell wonderful!
Au Gratin Potatoes- Assemble ahead and have in oven
Asparagus- steamed with butter and sprinkled with parmesan cheese. Can be prepared ahead and kept warm.
Green salad- more than just lettuce and tomatoes? Elevate! Try cucumbers, avocado, crouton, radishes
Rolls and sliced breads and butter

Dinner Parties

Don't be intimidated! The easiest way is to go is Family style. Put big bowls of food on the table and let everyone help themselves! Have beautiful tables all set with silverware, candles, a smaller centerpiece, and let everyone enjoy each other!

Here are some inspired menus submitted by my students:

Menu for New Year's Reunion Dinner for Eight
Courtesy of Diana Walters

Oven roasted pork (Boston Butt) roasted on top of thick layer of sweet onions. Top covered in thick onion slices. Lots of salt and pepper.
Baked sauerkraut, mix regular and Bavarian style. Add to roaster with all juice.
German potato salad
Fresh green salad with tomato, cucumber, kalamata olives, yellow bell pepper, olive oil and lemon dressing
Flourless chocolate torte or fruit pie

Super Bowl Party Menu
Courtesy of Brenda Edwards

Deviled eggs
Chicken Wings
Nachos
Artichoke Spinach Dip
Buffalo Chicken Dip
Pepperoni Pizza Casserole
Sub Sandwich
Potato Skins
Ham and cheese sliders
Marshmallow crispy treats
Football cake
Brownie batter dip
Jell-O shots
Punch

Menu for my "You're an Angel" Dessert Holiday Party
Courtesy of Vicki Escueda

Angel food cake
Vanilla Ice Cream and strawberry or cherry sauce
Peppermint Ice Cream
Whipped Cream
Devil's Food Cake
Chocolate Ice Cream and Chocolate Sauce
Assorted Nuts
Wine, Dessert Liqueurs
Coffee
Non-Alcoholic Punch

VEAPS & Volumes Christmas Party

Champagne with garnishes of frozen cranberries
Cream Cheese and chives with pecan bites
Spinach and blue cheese stuffed mushrooms
Roasted Pork loin with Dijon mustard and rosemary sauce
Potatoes Au Gratin
Steamed green beans
Salad of Boston lettuce, pecans, beets, goat cheese in light vinaigrette
Vanilla ice cream topped with chocolate sauce and accented with raspberries and mint sprigs
Spring water and assorted wines

Menu for Thanksgiving with Linda, Dawn, Friends and Family
Courtesy of Linda Kramer

Appetizers (around the room): Assorted nut plates, veggies and fruit with dips, coconut chicken bites.

Open Bar: Alcoholic and non-alcoholic drinks

Main Course:
Sliced Roast Turkey, Cheesy mashed Potatoes, regular mashed potatoes, green bean casserole, stuffing, sliced and homemade cranberry sauce, peas, rolls and garlic butter
Sliced ham, sweet potatoes or yams in brown sugar glaze
Assorted salads and additional sides

Dessert: Coffee, tea, apple, pumpkin and pecan pies, carrot cake, banana bread, ice cream

Cozy Holiday Casual Dinner

Appetizers: Pinecone Cheese Ball, Raw vegetable wreath with creamy salsa dip

Drinks: Christmas sangria, beer, wine

Buffet: Creamy split pea soup, Roasted tomato basil soup, Parmesan cheese straws, Monte Cristo sliders, mixed greens with pears and cranberries salad

Dessert: Platter of Christmas cookies and candies

LET'S TALK ABOUT CHEESE!

A variety of cheeses can act as workhorses in entertaining. Cheese is versatile when paired with fruit, nuts, and wines. It can be incorporated into many successful main dishes, and even desserts. Have a go-to cheese course for each type of party. Taste and become familiar with different cheeses before you serve them. Make sure you love what you serve and have fun with a variety. See the Appendix and Glossary of Cheeses in this book.

Cheeses are often served on a cheese board which can be wood, porcelain, or marble.

To slice soft cheese, use a cheese slicer with a wire. For hard cheeses, use a cheese scraper or grater. Good tools are very important!

Basic Cheese Guidelines

If you are serving cheese before dinner, choose lighter cheeses such as herb-coated goat cheese or fresh mozzarella.

If you are serving cheese after dinner, then you go one of two ways: serve just one rich and creamy cheese such as the easy to find triple-creme cheese called St. Andre- or go for full flavored cheeses like Manchego, cheddar, aged gouda, and/or blue cheeses.

Think of a theme – perhaps you can focus on the cheeses of the United States or even a specific region within the U.S. or Spain, Italy, or France. That automatically narrows the field.

Serving Cheese

- Be sure to serve cheese at room temperature. To do this, take the cheese out of the refrigerator at least one hour ahead of serving time.
- Serve before-dinner cheeses with relatively savory accompaniments such as olives, prosciutto, nuts, and/or chutney.
- Serve after-dinner cheeses with sweet accompaniments such as jams, honey, dried fruit, and toasted nuts.

Cheese Portions

If you are serving cheese as an appetizer, plan on 1 or 2 ounces of each cheese per person

If you are serving the cheese as an after-dinner cheese course, figure 1 to 1-1/2 ounces of each cheese per person.

Once you have determined the above, you'll need to decide how many cheeses to buy. Usually, one really great cheese is enough because it is so satisfying that it becomes a conversation piece. The exception is when cheese is the centerpiece of your party. In that case, you'll need at least three and probably five or six different cheeses. However, most of the time, serving three cheeses is adequate. That way you won't overwhelm your guests with too many choices.

Always taste any cheese before you serve it to your guests and make sure they go together with whatever else you are serving.

Ways to Use Cheese

Meat and Cheese Platter - Best done on a round platter or tray. This is a great staple because it can be put together the day before.

- Place large round doily on bottom of tray.
- Place individual thinly sliced meats (such as salami and/or ham) around the edge of the tray.
- Place individual slices of cheese sliced thin (such as Swiss and Cheddar) around the inner edge of the meat, slightly overlapping the first circle. Sargento brand has ultra-thin sliced Swiss and Cheddar that works very well.
- Keep going in circles with alternates of cheese or meat until there is a small circle in the middle.
- If you have a large group or a long party ahead, you can do another layer on top of the bottom layer.
- Place a bunch of parsley in the middle with some cherry tomatoes.
- Put a basket of crackers next to the round platter for a great go-to in cocktail parties or any kind of party.

Charcuterie

A great deal has been made about this artistic presentation of wonderful foods with a new book written by Marco Nicoli, *Charcuterie Boards* available on Amazon. A charcuterie board can be small and impressive with any number of ingredients; primarily different cheese, fruit, nuts, and sausage or salami beautifully presented. If the cheese is to be sliced, make sure there is enough room and cheese slicers for your guests to do so

Cheese Dips

Always good with crackers, chips, breads or even vegetables. Find a good cheese dip as your go-to. Great for cocktail parties and potlucks. Many cheese dips incorporate cream cheese because it is easy to spread and is usually served at near room temperature. There are some good commercial spreads like Boursin. Hot cheese dips are always impressive and can be assembled the day before and warmed before the party.

Main Dishes

Cheese is an ingredient for dishes from all over the world. Many cheeses are available already shredded and are often mixed with other cheeses. Find a brand that works for you in taste and ability to melt well. This is a real time-saver, and often a main dish casserole can be assembled the day before and warmed just before the event.

How about a Mac and Cheese Buffet dish? Make a killer Mac and Cheese and have different toppings for your guests to use like ham, bacon, diced tomato . . . use your imagination!

Desserts

I love serving a good cheese with fruit for dessert. It reminds me of trips to Europe. Cheesecake is always a favorite and can be made ahead of time. Think about mini cheesecakes as hostess gifts to send home with your guests! Make a double batch with a large cheesecake for your party and save the mini cheesecakes for them to take home.

Platters

Not boring at all, and always a crowd pleaser. Your go-to cheese platter should be cheeses that you love and feel confident serving.

SECRETS OF STRESS-FREE ENTERTAINING

- Always do a taste test before your party.
- Cheese should be served at room temperature, so make sure it has time to breathe before your party.

Provide two or three kinds of complimentary cheese, some crackers, a bunch of grapes, and a sliced apple . . .DONE! Ultimate finger food. Great for a cocktail party.

Before you get started, here's what to consider:

- How many people are you serving?"
- Are you serving cheese before dinner or as an after-dinner cheese course?
- Are there any cheeses you definitely want to include or maybe avoid?
- What is your budget?

Arranging Your Cheese Platter

- Never crowd your cheese platters. If you do, you are likely to find your knuckle in one cheese while attempting to cut the one you're really after.
- Offer a different knife with each cheese. If you cut all the cheeses with just one knife, they will start tasting like each other.
- Serve slices of a baguette or crackers in a separate basket or bowl.
- Choose plain (sourdough or French) bread or neutral crackers. Flavored breads such as ones with sesame seeds, or garlic and herbed crackers, tend to overwhelm the flavors of cheeses. The exceptions are breads containing walnuts, dried fruit, or olives. These all compliment a cheese.
- As a dessert, serve the cheeses either on one or more platters, or plate them individually. The latter method works particularly well if you are serving cheeses after dinner. Each person should be served their own plate, and best of all, you get to prepare the cheese course *before* your guests arrive, leaving one less last-minute thing to do. The plates can sit at room temperature, lightly covered, for a couple of hours without harming the cheese unless

your kitchen is particularly warm. In that case, keep them refrigerated until an hour before serving time.

How about a cheese tasting party?
Begin with some nice wines, then serve fruit such as sliced apples and grapes, and some assorted crackers or a sliced baguette of bread. This is also great to schedule before going out in the afternoon or dinner. Do some research about the cheeses you are serving and share the information with your guests. Refer to the Appendix on the Glossary of Cheeses in the back of this book and you will sound like a true cheese expert!

Here are several idea suggestions:

- Choose **one cheese made with each type of dairy**: Cow, goat, or sheep's milk.
- Choose **cheeses all made with one type of milk**, such as sheep's milk. Doing that is a great way to learn about different styles of cheese within one milk category.
- Select different **cheeses within the same family of cheeses**. Examples of this would be three or four styles of soft-ripened cheeses such as Brie and Camembert and any other cheeses that have a similar white downy-like rind. Or you can select a few distinct styles of blue cheese. This is a great way to learn how similar cheeses differ sometimes widely in flavor.
- Choose **cheeses with different textures**. Go for a soft and creamy cheese such as Brie (or a similar artisan -style cheese made in your area); a firmer style cheese such as cheddar (preferably farmhouse), gouda or Gruyere; and a hard grating style cheese like Parmigiano-Reggiano.

THE ESSENTIAL GOUGÉRES

These amazing little morsels of magic are wonderful for breakfast, lunch, dinner, snacks, or appetizers. They absolutely melt in your mouth and are addictive. We used to make these in our catering days, and they were always a star item. Try and make them, no matter what your skill set. It's not a difficult recipe. It is easy to master but will take a little technique. However, it will always impress your guests who may ask if you trained at the Cordon Bleu!

The easiest way to describe "gougéres" is to call them cheese puffs. Gougéres are a classic dough, called Pâte á Choux, only with cheese added. Pâte á Choux is the recipe you would use for sweet cream puffs or profiteroles. To make a gougére, simply fold in a fair amount of grated cheese. Then choose a cheese you like; use several to give each a different taste treat. You can use Gruyere, Emmenthal, extra sharp Cheddar, or you can try a smoked cheese. Pair with Champagne, wine, or an aperitif for a perfect simple appetizer.

It's a good idea to make several batches and freeze them. Refer below for instructions on best results.

Pâte á Choux

1/2 Cup whole milk
1/2 Cup water
8 tbsp. (1 stick) unsalted butter, cut into 4 pieces
1/2 teaspoon salt
1 Cup all-purpose Flour
5 large eggs, at room temperature

For gougéres
1-1/2 Cups coarsely grated cheese, such as Gruyere or Cheddar (approx. 6 oz.)

Position racks to divide oven into thirds and preheat to 425 degrees F. Line baking sheets with silicone baking mats or parchment paper.
Bring the milk, water, butter, and salt to a rapid boil in a heavy-bottomed medium saucepan over high heat. Add the flour all at once, lower the heat to medium-low, and immediately start stirring energetically with a wooden spoon or heavy whisk. The dough will come together, and a light coating or

crust will form on the bottom of the pan. Keep stirring with vigor for another minute or two to dry the dough. The dough should now be smooth.

Turn the dough into the bowl of a mixer fitted with the paddle attachment or into a bowl that can used for mixing with a hand mixer or a wood spoon with lots of elbow grease. Let the dough sit for a minute then add the eggs one by one and continue beating until the dough is thick and shiny. Make sure each egg is completely incorporated before adding the next, and don't be concerned if the dough separates—by the time the last egg goes in, the dough will come together again. Beat in the grated cheese.

Once the dough is made, it should be spooned immediately unto the baking sheets.

Using about 1 tablespoon of dough for each gougére, drop the dough from the spoon onto the lined baking sheets, leaving about 2 inches of puff space between the mounds.
Slide the baking sheets into the oven and immediately turn the oven temperature down to 375 degrees F.

Bake for 12 minutes, then rotate pans from front to back and top to bottom. Continue baking until the gougéres are golden, firm, and yes, puffed, about another 12 to 15 minutes or so. Serve warm, or transfer to racks to cool. Enjoy warm or at room temperature.

Storing and Freezing
The best way to store gougéres is to shape the dough, freeze the mounds on a baking sheet, and then, when they are solid, lift them off the sheet and pack them airtight in plastic bags. Bake them straight from the freezer - no need to defrost - just give them another minute or two in the oven. Leftover puffs can be kept at room temperature overnight and reheated in a 350 degrees F. oven, or they can be frozen and reheated before serving.

Change it Up
The beauty of mastering this recipe is that it is so versatile and perfect for entertaining.

Follow the recipe but delete the cheese. Then you will have a basic Pâte á Choux.

Make small puffs and stuff with egg salad, chicken salad, or shrimp salad for impressive appetizers. Wait until the puffs cool and then stuff.

You can make small puffs and stuff them with whipped cream and topped with chocolate. Or make larger puffs and stuff with custard or pudding. Great for dessert, breakfast, or a brunch.

In the back of this book is a section of additional cheese recipes. There are so many, and I urge you to try them. Cheese truly is the workhorse in extraordinary party venues!

THE IMPORTANCE OF TABLETOP TENTS

Once you are sure of your menu, it is a good time to create your Menu Tents. I really believe in them. I like to have tents listing ingredients of each dish and placed next to each one I am serving. With so many allergies and food sensitivities, my guests should know what they are eating for their own safety and well-being. If it is a Potluck, ask what the ingredients are in each dish people are bringing, and explain to the contributors why you are asking for a list of the ingredients. Be consistent in making tents for each dish. It only needs to be index-sized cardstock folded in half to create a self-standing "tent" card with ingredients printed or typed. Put the title of the dish at the top. You can include the name of the contributing chef if it's for a Potluck. Blank note cards are a good size. You can even decorate the tents consistent with your theme, just for fun.

In part 2 of Chapter 5, we will learn how to use the Master Template.

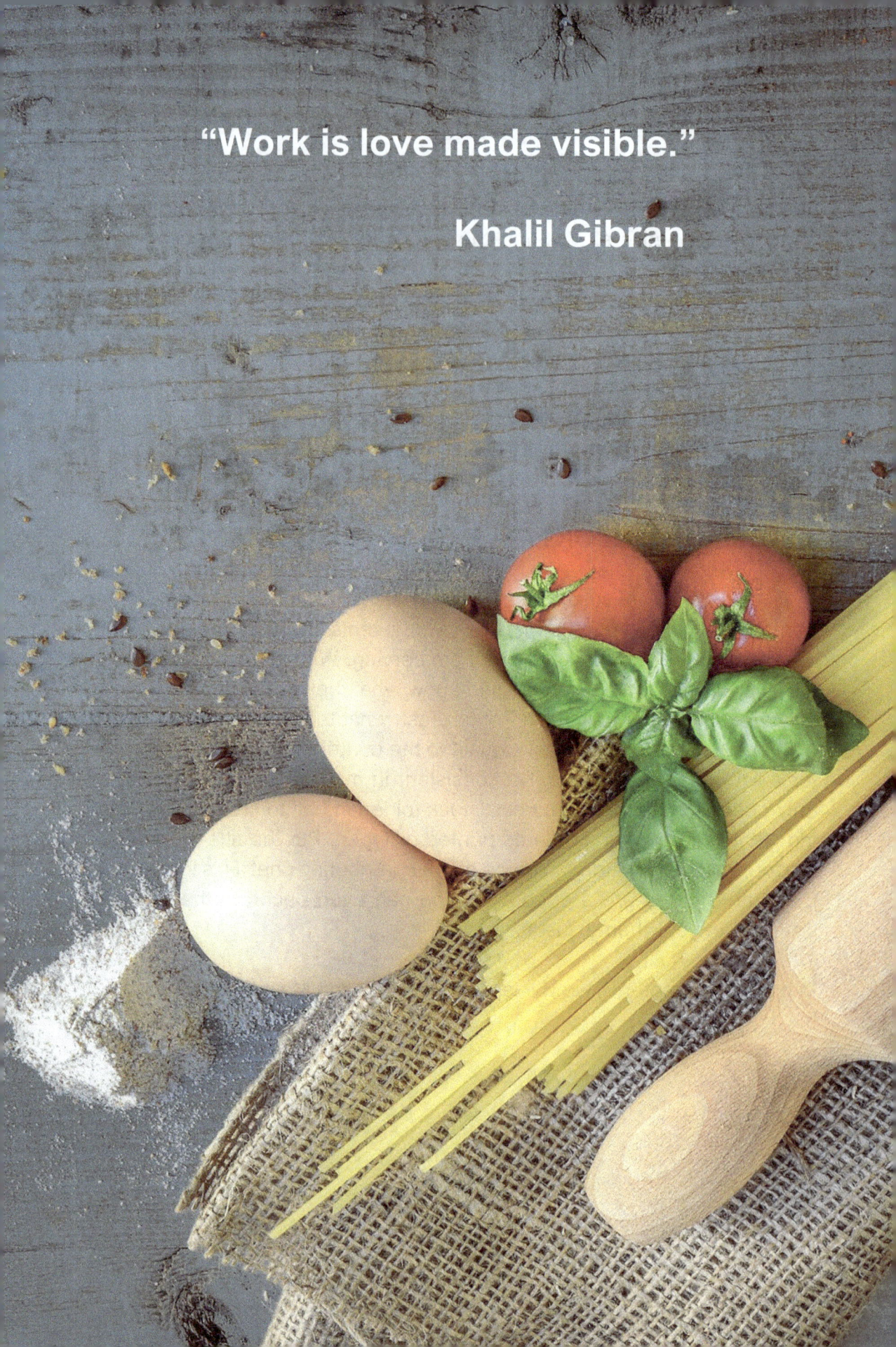

Chapter 5
WEEK THREE
All About Templates

PART TWO

THE MASTER TEMPLATE

This is probably the most valuable part of this entire book. This template can guide you in putting together any party, any size, and any kind. Everything you need to put your party together will be organized with your 2 step Template. The Template will provide all the information that you need to shop, prepare, cook, and serve the food for your party. Page One of the Template will have your shopping lists and menu in one place. The Master Template Blueprint will detail every aspect of your food preparation for your party.

    The first thing you will do is to make your own Master Template. Use a sharpened pencil with an eraser. You will also need a ruler and a few pages of unlined binder paper. Make lots of copies of page one and page two.

THE MASTER TEMPLATE

The Shopping List Tool

MENU

List ingredients

1. _____
2. _____
3. _____
4. _____
5. _____
6. _____
7. _____

INITIAL SHOPPING LIST (Up to Two Weeks Ahead)

(**Examples:** canned goods, frozen goods, nuts, olives, items that last longer than one week. Also toothpicks, plastic wrap ziplock bags, foil, alcohol, juices, paper products. This list should be the largest shopping trip.)

_____
_____
_____
_____
_____
_____
_____

FINAL SHOPPING LIST (Two Days Before the Event)

(**Examples:** Items that should be fresh – fruits and vegetables, dairy, crackers, cheese, meats. Also include curly parsley, cherry tomatoes, grapes and romaine lettuce for plate presentations and trays.)

_____
_____
_____
_____
_____
_____
_____

The Preparation List Tool

The Master Template (continued)

COLD DISH	SERVED IN	SERVING TOOL	PREPARE	PREP TIME	PLATE		CHECK OFF

HOT DISH	SERVED IN	SERVING TOOL	PREPARE	PREP TIME	STOVE	OVEN TEMP/TIME	CHECK OFF

HOW TO USE THE MASTER TEMPLATE

Write small and include as much detail as you can about each menu item. Always use pencil. Assemble the recipes of your menu items.

It's time to commit to your final menu. This will be an opportunity to judge if you have balance in your choices. Too many hot dishes? Too many cold? Too many salty dishes? Too many dishes requiring last-minute preparation. This will show any weakness in your menu choices. Assemble the recipes of the dishes you will be serving. If it's a potluck and people are bringing dishes, make sure to include them on your final menu.

Check your pantry and freezer to make sure you don't already have something you need. We're all guilty about not knowing everything on our shelves. List your menu items under Menu at the top of page 1. I have found seven items to be the magic number for most buffets.

Go to the first menu item and designate each ingredient under the Initial Shopping List or Final Shopping List on page 1.

Items under the Initial Shopping List

These ingredients will be those that can be purchased ahead of time like canned goods, frozen goods, nuts, olives, and items that will last longer than a week. Include your bar needs in the Initial Shopping trip. Your Initial Shopping List should also include toothpicks, Saran Wrap, zip lock bags, foil, alcohol, juices, paper products. The goal should be that your Initial Shopping Trip is the largest.

Items for the Final Shopping List should be items that you want to be the freshest like fruits and vegetables, dairy, crackers, cheese, and meat. Always include curly parsley, cherry tomatoes, grapes, and Romaine lettuce for best presentation on your trays.

Now go to page two and fill out the Master Template Blueprint

- List each menu item under Hot Dish or Cold Dish.
- Decide what each dish will be served in. A tray? A bowl?
- What Serving Tool will the dish need? Spoon? Tongs?

- What is involved in the preparation? Can you prepare it the day before? The week before? Can it be frozen?
- What is the preparation time? Include all the details.
- When can you plate your dish? Can you plate it the day before, and keep it in the refrigerator? Do you need to plate it the morning of the event? Anything you can do ahead of time is a plus.
- For those hot dishes, decide if you need the stovetop or the oven. If it is a stovetop item, what pot will it be cooked in? If it is going in the oven, what temperature should the oven be set? It's best to limit your oven items to only one or two. If you have multiple items to go in the oven, different cooking temperatures could become difficult.
- Keep in mind the number of items that will require your stovetop. If you only have four burners and have five items that need to be heated up, it will not work well. Now is the time to make that adjustment to your menu.

Once you have completed these two pages, you can really evaluate your menu choices. If you need to change something, now is the time to do it!

If you are hosting a potluck where your friends will be bringing items, this is the week to find out what they are bringing. Get a list of the ingredients of what they are bringing so that you include it with your tents. Add their items to your master menu and separate it from those items you are providing.

LET'S GET SOME PRACTICE WITH THE TEMPLATES!

Below we will go through an exercise using one of my favorite buffet menus which is a "quick and easy" one for me. It's always well received, has a good rhythm in preparation, and is balanced with hot and cold items. Following the recipes and menu, we will fill out the Master templates for Shopping and Preparation.

Recipes and Menu for Super Easy Party

Ham Rollups

Can of asparagus full stalks (Green Giant is best)
Original cream cheese (1 container does full package of ham)
Packaged Sliced Ham (Publix prepackaged is a very good thickness)

Separate ham slices on cutting board. Spread softened cream cheese on each slice of ham. Place 1 long stalk of asparagus at the end. Roll up and package separately in saran wrap. Chill for several hours (or overnight.) Slice in 1-inch slices with sharp knife. Each ham rollup makes about 4 pinwheels. Place on serving dish. Can use toothpick to secure although the cream cheese is like the "glue" holding it together very well. They look like little pinwheels when sliced.

Salami and Cheese Tray

Take sliced salami and work around the tray overlapping each piece. Cut the sliced cheese (a yellow and a white cheese best) diagonally. Arrange on inside of salami working around tray.

Easy to stack depending on number of guests. Put some parsley and grape tomatoes in the middle of the tray.

Veggie Tray

Cut into easy-to-eat pieces carrots, celery, red pepper, cucumber, whatever you like. Arrange on tray and place ramekin with Hidden Valley Ranch dressing for dipping.

Deviled Eggs

Cook eggs. Cool. Shell and cut in half and separate yolk. Mash yolks and make your favorite recipe using mayonnaise, mustard, whatever. Try to find a special deviled egg dish for serving. You can sprinkle a little paprika on top for color.

Meatballs in Chili Sauce

Frozen meatballs are best. Dump a full bottle of Chili Sauce (Heinz best) into a saucepan and warm up meatballs according to directions. Put in chafing Dish or crock pot. Serve with toothpicks.

Hot Artichoke dip with either crackers or bread

14 oz. can of artichoke hearts chopped
1 Cup parmesan cheese (grated works fine)
1 Cup mayonnaise

Drain artichoke hearts and add mayo and cheese. Can be assembled day before. Cook in 350-degree oven for 20 minutes. It will be very hot so let cool a bit before serving.

I like to cook in an oven safe au gratin dish, serve on tray and surround with either crackers or chunks of good bread with a crunchy crust (French bread ideal). If using bread best to provide knife. You can also serve it in a hollowed out round loaf of French bread after cooking. (do not cook bread)

Little Smokies in Barbecue sauce

Put full bottle of barbecue sauce (I like Heinz original) in saucepan and package of little smokies or little hot dogs.
Heat until warm and serve in chafing dish or crock pot. Serve with toothpicks.

PRACTICE TEMPLATE EXERCISE

Menu
Ham Roll Ups
Salami and Cheese
Veggie Tray
Deviled Eggs
Meatballs in Chili Sauce
Little Smokies in Barbecue Sauce
Artichoke Dip with Crackers or Bread

Initial Shopping List (up to 2 weeks ahead)
Check supplies of toothpicks, foil, Saran Wrap, bags
Canned asparagus (long spears)
Mustard
Hidden Valley Ranch Dressing
2 bottles chili sauce
Large mayonnaise
Canned artichoke hearts
Frozen meatballs
Parmesan cheese
2 Bottles barbecue sauce
Package of little smokies
Canned nuts
Green olives for Martinis

Final Shopping List (2 days before event)
<u>Fresh fruit and veggies</u>: Lemons, limes, parsley, cherry tomatoes, grapes, Romaine lettuce, carrots, celery, red peppers, cucumbers.
<u>Meats/ Cheeses/ Dairy</u>: Package sliced ham
1 package cream cheese, sliced salami, sliced cheddar cheese, sliced Swiss cheese, eggs, breads: crackers, small baguette, thin breadsticks

 From the information that has been compiled and organized, we've learned all kinds of valuable information needed to stay organized, prepared, and stress-free!
 You learned how many trays are needed, what serve ware is necessary, how many bowls are needed, how many items need to go on the stovetop, what to put on two complete shopping lists, and what to buy. The practice template teaches us lots of useful information in the planning of this party.

USING THE MASTER TEMPLATE

The Shopping List Tool

MENU

1. **Ham Roll-Ups** – ham, asparagus, cream cheese
2. **Trays** – salami, sliced cheese
3. **Veggie Tray** – carrots, celery, zucchini, red pepper
4. **Deviled Eggs** – eggs, mayo, mustard
5. **Meatballs** – frozen meatballs, chili sauce
6. **Artichoke Dip** – artichokes, Parmesan cheese, mayo
7. **Smokies** – smokies sausages, barbeque sauce

INITIAL SHOPPING LIST (Up to Two Weeks Ahead)

(**Examples**: canned goods, frozen goods, nuts, olives, items that last longer than one week. Also toothpicks, plastic wrap zip lock bags, foil, alcohol, juices, and paper products. This list should be the largest shopping trip.)

1. Can asparagus
2. Can artichokes
3. Frozen meatballs
4. Barbeque sauce
5. Grated Parmesan cheese
6. Mayonnaise smokies sausages
7. Mustard

FINAL SHOPPING LIST (Two Days Before the Event)

(**Examples:** Items that should be fresh – fruits and vegetables, dairy, crackers, cheese, meats. Also include curly parsley, cherry tomatoes, grapes and romaine lettuce for plate presentations and trays.)

1. Sliced ham
2. Cream cheese
3. Sliced salami
4. Sliced cheese
5. Eggs
6. Zucchini
7. Red pepper
8. Celery
9. Carrot

Sample: How to Use the Master Template

The Master Template (Page 2)

COLD DISH	SERVED IN	SERVING TOOL	PREPARE	PREP TIME	PLATE		CHECK OFF
Ham Roll-Ups	Tray	Toothpicks	Day Before	45 min.	Day Before		
Salami and Cheese	Tray	Tongs/Fork	Day Before	30 min.	Day Before		
Veggie Tray	Tray/Bowl for Dip	None	Prepare 2 days ahead	1 hour	Day Before		
Deviled Eggs	Deviled Egg Platter	Tongs	Cook eggs 2 days ahead	50 min.	Day Before		
HOT DISH	SERVED IN	SERVING TOOL	PREPARE	PREP TIME	STOVE	OVEN TEMP/ TIME	CHECK OFF
Meatballs/Chili Sauce	Chafing Dish	Spoon	Day of Party	30 min. 20 min.	Stovetop Crockpot		
Artichoke Dip	Ovenproof dip dish	None	Day Before	20 min.		20 min. at 350 degrees	
Smokies in BBQ Sauce	Chafing dish	Toothpicks	Day of Party	20 min.	Warm in saucepan	crockpot	

In Summary:

Two Days Before:
- Final shopping
- Cook eggs
- Clean Veggies

Day Before:
- Assemble ham roll-ups, cut and plate
- Do salami and cheese trays
- Make deviled eggs and plate
- Assemble veggie tray
- Make artichoke dip; do not cook until the next day

Day of:
- Meatballs
- Smokies
- Cook artichoke dip

SUMMARY OF WEEK THREE

This was a very busy week. We've covered:
- Hostess gifts ready
- Checked inventory
- Planned and stocked the bar
- Party theme and decorations purchased
- Reservations followed-up
- Nailed down all details
- Mastered the Master Template
- Committed to your final menu.

Your lists are organized with every detail. You are definitely coming down the home stretch.

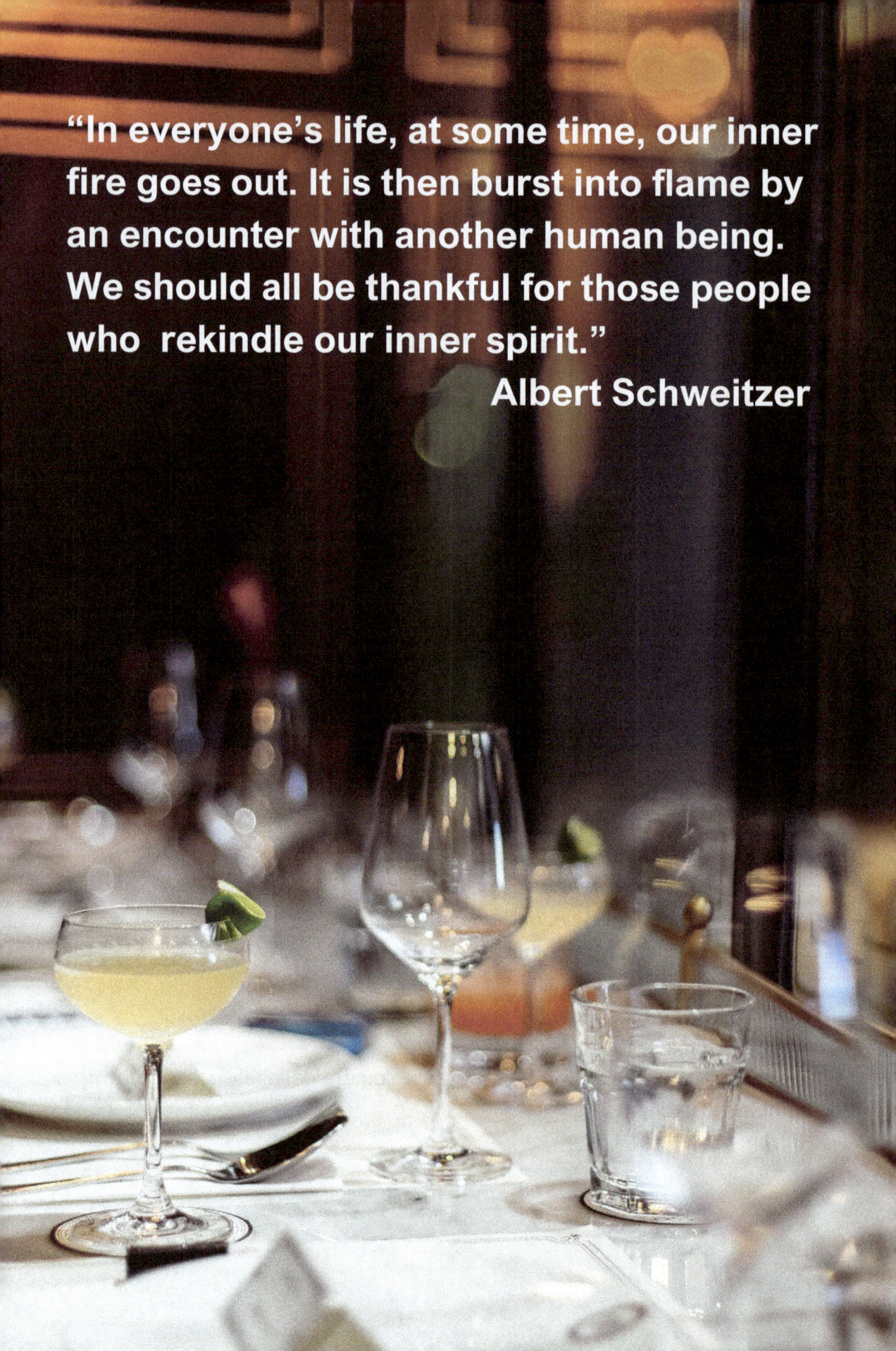

"In everyone's life, at some time, our inner fire goes out. It is then burst into flame by an encounter with another human being. We should all be thankful for those people who rekindle our inner spirit."

Albert Schweitzer

Chapter 6
WEEK FOUR
Almost Party Time

THE FINAL COUNTDOWN

You've been working hard, and the finish line is in sight! Go through your lists, edit items still to be done, and focus on this very important last week. Because you've been planning and working ahead, the last week shouldn't be too difficult.

- **Parking** Notify neighbors of the event and address any parking issues. Better yet, invite your neighbors! If not, take over a bottle of wine after the event, especially if they've been inconvenienced in any way with parking or noise.
- **Decorating** Finish decorating the house with all the finishing touches for your party.
- **Cleaning** Have any house cleaning completed in the beginning of the week. You might schedule the cleaners to come back *after* your party, too!
- **Ice** Continue bagging ice.
- **RSVP's** Follow up on all RSVP's and get a final count of the number of guests. Don't be shy! Knowing the count is very important.

- **Hostess Gifts** Wrap and complete.
- **Silverware** Wrap in napkins and tie with ribbon or napkin rings.
- **Lights** Hang party lights both inside and outside. Design your complete lighting plan.
- **Frozen Items** Make sure all frozen make-ahead items are in the freezer

Here is an Example of Where You Could Be in Your Planning

Joan's Magical Christmas Party

Here is a wonderful holiday party plan written by one of my students, Joan Reece, during one of my classes. She planned a large holiday buffet brunch that sounds delightful! She has a gift for helping us visualize exactly what she wants to achieve. When you can get to this point of having a mental picture of your party and can fill in the details, as she did, you will have complete confidence in what you have planned and created. Then you can truly relax and enjoy your own party!

Joan organized her party into three parts:

1. Room Set-up- giving a visual description of what her guests will see, feel, smell, and hear as they open the door to her party.
2. Food Set up—Explanation of how the food and drinks will be set out and/or served.
3. Menu-Planning: Thoughtful and balanced

She begins:

"My party will be a Christmas morning Brunch for eight to 12 couples. It will be a drop-in type of event from 9:30 to 11:30 Am on Christmas morning. The food will be served buffet-style. There will be multiple places to sit, eat, and visit via two large tables which will each accommodate eight people, and our large seating area in the living room, which can seat an additional 11 people. While this will be a warm and casual event, it will be festive and special, and filled with holiday cheer!

Room Set-Up

A tall white tree with white lights will be visible through the double-sized arched front window as you walk up to our front door. A sparkly wreath made of small shiny silver balls will sparkle on our dark-colored front door. Cone-shaped lighted topiaries will stand on each side of the door, beckoning you to enter.

As you enter, a tasteful number of red poinsettias and Christmas treasures will be strategically placed throughout. Colorful Christmas throw cushions will welcome you to our large sectional sofa. The electric fireplace in our stone wall will be burning brightly, and instrumental Christmas music will be softly playing in the background.

As you walk into our living room, a seven-and-a-half-foot holiday tree situated on our newly enclosed lanai will be partially visible. The tree will be decorated with white lights and red, white, and silver ornaments. The tree will be fully visible from the kitchen and nook area through the angled window to the lanai, and fully visible from the large farmhouse table on the left end of the lanai.

The large farmhouse table, which can seat eight people, will be simply decorated down the center with a sprinkling of either holly and red berries or small fir branches with red berries. A few polished Wallace heirloom ornaments with a red velvet ribbon tied through the hoop will be resting among the greenery. At the opposite end of the lanai, tucked away among the UGA collectibles, a pencil tree will be decorated with Georgia Bulldog football ornaments. "Ugh," our three-foot-tall bulldog statue will be standing by the tree wearing a Santa Hat and holding a lighted strand of holly.

Outside the lanai, red poinsettias, red amaryllis flowers, and our large Christmas cactus, will be blooming among the palms, shrubs, and ferns. For anyone who prefers to take their food outside in the garden, just outside the lanai under the pergola is a large round counter height stone top table that will seat eight people. It will have a woodsy centerpiece utilizing the red and green color theme found all around.

Food Set-Up

Back in the '80's, while living in what was then West Germany, I purchased a large number of party dishes in a Christmas pattern. They have a shiny red background, with a green tree decorated with white candles and stars. I still have three dozen mugs, about that many small plates and multiple serving dishes. Since it is festive and something a little different, I will use these dishes.

I also have enough silver-plated silverware to cover a group of this size, so I will polish and use it. And, of course, champagne glasses for the mimosas.

The food will be set up on the bar and our nook table. Serving bowls and platters will either be the same pattern as the mugs and plates or will be solid white or clear glass.

There will be a coffee, hot tea, and hot chocolate station set up in one area of the kitchen. Another area will be set up for making mimosas on demand. Pitchers of orange and apple juice will also be at the mimosa area.

Menu Planning

My festive brunch menu is still under construction. I am more of a gatherer than a cook or baker. I do have a few brunch staples that I know will be on the menu. I would like to find festive holiday versions of those items. Since it will be a brunch, not just breakfast, I would like to have a festive Charcuterie board. I'm so excited that we will be learning about those in class. Here are some of my menu ideas:

- Breakfast casserole
- Boiled eggs
- Bacon/ ham slices
- Croissants
- Fruit tray
- Charcuterie board or a meat and cheese platter
- Couple types of sweet bread
- Gingerbread cookies
- Decorated sugar cookies.

Thank you, Joan!

Visualizing your party will add to your self-confidence and that will help you enjoy your own party. This one sounds like so much fun!

The countdown . . . You've got this!

Four Days Before Event

- **Coats** Decide where coats and purses will go.
- **Furniture** Set up the bar and move furniture around as needed. Make sure your guests can move freely throughout your house. Make sure there are no cords or rugs guests can trip over.
- **Clean up** Decide on where the trash will go. Plan for who will do cleaning and take full bags of trash out to the garage during the event? Enlist any help you can with cleaning up after your guests go home. I prefer to keep the kitchen under control while people are there, without taking time away from my guests. It's a bit of a balancing act. Defer the majority of clean-up until after your guests leave. It's okay to ask a very close friend to stay and help, if you are tired. Try and get as much cleaned up before you go to bed as there is nothing worse than waking up to a mess.
- **Bar** Do preliminary set up of the bar area with napkins, stir sticks, and miscellaneous items. Set out containers for everything! Lemons, limes, celery. Set out as much as possible beforehand other than ice. Then cross them off the list!

Three Days Before Event:

- **Flowers** Buy and arrange flowers for the house and centerpieces, keeping with your colors and theme. I've always felt that orchids are best for my parties as they last for weeks or even months after the event with only minimal care. If buying fresh flowers, look for buds when you purchase! With Florida heat, they will open quickly. Change water one day before the party.
- **Centerpieces** If not flowers, complete whatever arrangements you are planning to use. Finish the task and cross it off your list! Make it wonderful and inspiring with creative finishing touches.
- **Medicine Chest** Remove any prescription medications from your bathroom, especially if there are people coming to your party that you don't know well. I know it may sound extreme, but people will snoop. They will never admit it, but many will open your medicine cabinet and check out what's inside. Believe it. People do it!

- **Expensive Jewelry and Cash** Remove and secure any expensive jewelry and cash you keep in the house. You might never think one of your guests would put something in their pocket. As ugly as it seems, don't provide any temptation.
- **Ice** Continue bagging ice!

Two Days Before Event:

- **Final Shopping Day!** If you have a great deal of food prep, shop three days before your party. Schedule your shopping trip early in the day. You should have already made your initial shopping during Week 3, so this day's trip should include fresh fruits, vegetables, meats, and perishables.
- **Food Preparation**
  1. Start washing, slicing and dicing. Easiest way is with a colander in the sink. Have small and large zip lock bags available for storage in the refrigerator.
  2. Wash and peel carrots, celery, radishes, raw peppers, and more. Cut in desired pieces, wrap in a moistened paper towel, and put into plastic containers with labels.
  3. Wash parsley and lettuce then wrap in wet paper towels and store in a baggie.
  4. Cut limes and lemons and put into small zip lock bags.
  5. Cut up any ingredients that are needed for a casserole.
  6. Marinate any meats and cover in plastic.
  7. Take out anything that needs to begin defrosting and move it to the refrigerator.
- **Assembly** This is an exciting part of your plan where you will begin to see how everything is coming together. Pull out table settings, plates, serving dishes, serving utensils, and other serving items. If it's a buffet or potluck, begin spacing things out on your counter or table. Put a piece of masking tape on the bottom of plates and trays to designate what is being served on that plate. Any decision made ahead of time, reduces stress at the last minute. Check your list and make sure you have included everything.
- **Refrigerator Space** Your primary refrigerator space may start becoming an issue. Some people have an additional refrigerator

in the garage used to chill beverages. If you have one, it can be handy for additional food storage when you entertain. When buying plastic containers, buy several of the same size which you can stack. Label everything and organize containers so you can find them quickly. Group like ingredients together or put ingredients that will be used later in the same area of the refrigerator. Keep in mind to make room for any additions you might have for the following day.

One Day Before Event:

- Go over absolutely everything you can beforehand. Set out serving pieces, set tables, place centerpieces. Make it like a trial run.
- Set up trash stations. Line the trash cans with plastic liners. Have lots of extras. I like to put about four new bags on the bottom of the container, then put an unfolded one on top. That way when it is full, just lift out the filled trash bag and a clean one will be right there to open. Anticipate where your guests will need to dump their trash. Have several locations, hopefully away from the kitchen flow. You don't want your guests having to hunt around with a dirty plate in hand trying to find a trash container under your sink while you are working there.
- Go over all preparations and lists. Leave a list next to your stove listing anything having to be cooked to keep you on schedule. Include item, cooking time, and temperature. Have a full menu list handy and easily available. There is nothing worse than forgetting to serve a dish that's still in the back of your refrigerator!
- Do as much final cooking and preparation as you can.
- Start your party with an empty dishwasher. Run the Dishwasher right before you go to bed the night before.
- Double check your list, have your party clothes pulled out, and ready. Then go to bed in peace. It's very important for you to get a good night's sleep. Set the alarm if you must. You have done all your prep work and planning. You have everything under control!

Remember lists are your friends

Day of Event

- Finish any cooking and make it an easy morning, if possible.
- Shower and layout your clothes.
- Pull out any food items that need to be at room temperature.
- Pull out any necessary pots and pans
- Preheat the oven
- Empty the dishwasher
- Put out items such as chips, nuts, and non-perishables.
- Have a written timetable and "cheat sheet" to keep you on track.
- Greet your guests
- Take lots of pictures!
- Enjoy yourself! Listen to the laughter! Let your friends delight at the work you've done to make your party so special. Pause when they arrive and have a toast!

HOW TO HANDLE HICCUPS

You have done the planning, made your lists, so everything should run flawlessly, right? Sometimes, unexpected things happen. Just go with it. Maybe you forgot something. Maybe some guests did not show up who said they would. Maybe you overcooked something. It happens. Let it go.

My mother once told me to always avoid talking about religion and politics in social situations. It is truer now than ever. If you overhear a conversation heading in that direction, shut it down immediately. Change the subject, ask for help, whatever you need to do to intervene. You'll be glad you did.

Another situation that used to get to me is the neighbor who wants to take control of your party. How should you handle it? Refer to your list. Is there anything that needs to get done right now? Get it done quickly, get ahead of yourself, then turn to your friend and say: "There's nothing much left to do right now. Why don't you come out with me and talk to (fill in the blank)?" Then YOU continue to enjoy your own party.

Lots of people ask if they can help which I appreciate and almost always say, "Thank you! Everything's good!." But sometimes there will be someone who simply INSISTS on getting involved. I want to scream: "Get out of my kitchen! I've got this!" However, here is my favorite coping skill which I have found works very well. In fact, it works for any kind of stress you may encounter during your party:

Go to your master bathroom and close the door. Close your eyes. Breathe deeply for four counts - breathe in four times and breathe out four times. Do this five times in a row. Then clear your mind and start speaking these affirmations slowly and calmly:

"I am a Party Warrior. Nothing can shake me! I've got this. Everyone will have a wonderful time! This is going to be a fabulous party that people will remember and positively talk about for a long time."

Check your makeup, comb your hair, and smile at yourself in the mirror. Return to your guests. You'll have a skip in your step.

THE PARTY'S OVER

You've included a time that the party will be ending on the Invitation. It's getting late and you're getting a bit tired. Sometimes, guests just don't want to leave. Awkward.

When it's time for your guests to leave, it's always a nice idea to make sure you give each of them something to take home with them. You can hope they recognize it as a signal that the party is over.

If you have multiple guests who want to extend the party, I will usually start cleaning up, hoping that gives a signal it's time to go. Some will say they want to stay and help at which point you can say: "You know, it's getting late. Why don't you go on home and get a good night's rest? And here's a little gift for you to take home."

Let them know it was great to see them, how much fun you had, and how much you appreciated them coming!

Clean Up

My personal preference is to put all the food away first. Have all the supplies you need including plastic bags, plastic containers, and plastic wrap set up and ready to go.

Separate dishes for the dishwasher and any items to be hand-washed. Load the dishwasher. Then take all the trash out, take everything down, hand wash what's needed, clean everything up, and put everything away. You can enlist help if you like. Use this as valuable time to talk about everything that happened at the party, what worked and what didn't. Be sure to laugh about what didn't go so well. And that's it.

You did it! Sleep well; I'm sure it was an overwhelming success! Remember: Don't schedule anything important to do the next day!

It would be healthier to sleep late, schedule a massage, and watch a favorite movie. My best advice: Don't plan on leaving for a trip the next day.

SUMMARY OF WEEK FOUR
Here's a quick checklist to refer to for the last week:

Four Days Before Event
Decide where the coats and purses will go, move any furniture, decide on clean up, set up your bar.

Three Days Before Event
Buy and arrange any flowers, get your centerpieces done, clean out your medicine chest, finish all shopping.

Two Days Before Event
Begin food prep and cooking. Pull out table setting, plates, serving dishes, trays, etc.

One Day Before Event
Do everything you can before the event. Label everything and do a few test runs in how the serving area is set up. Set up your table linens and set-up your tables.

Day of Event
Finish any cooking and make it as easy a day as possible. Shower and lay out your clothes. Pull out any food that needs to be at room temperature. Pull out any necessary pots and pans. Preheat the oven. Empty the dishwasher. Display the food. Have a list and cheat sheet by the stove. Try and take pictures of everything that is set up before guests arrive. Greet guests. Take lots of pictures of guests having fun. Enjoy yourself!

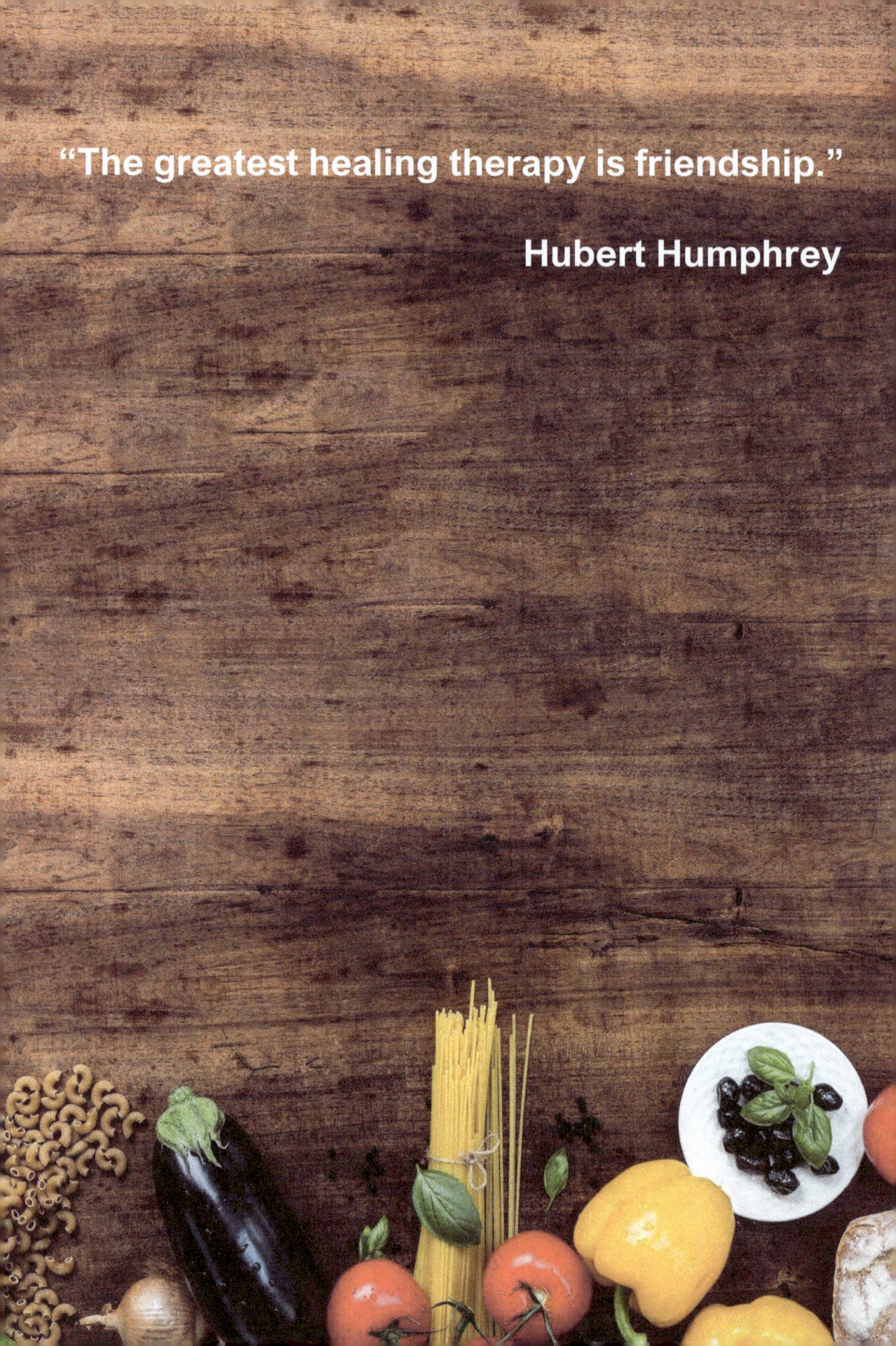
"The greatest healing therapy is friendship."

Hubert Humphrey

Chapter 7
Favorite Party Recipes

You may be a master chef, or you may hate the kitchen. This book will guide you in planning a party of any size whether you make food yourself or pick up the menu items at a store or from a restaurant. There are no judgements here! If you enjoy cooking, or would like to give it a try, this chapter has lots of wonderful recipes chosen for ease of preparation and number of ingredients.

BRUNCH

Brunch is one of my favorite parties! Easter and Christmas Mornings are perfect times for holiday celebrations; however, you can do a Brunch any time of the year. Many items can be cooked the day before and are well-received. Figure your prep time will require an earlier start, but the benefit is an early clean-up. Add some Bloody Mary's or Mimosas, and you have a memorable party. You might even have time for an afternoon nap!

Below is the menu I recently served to sixteen people for a memorable Easter Brunch. The weather was glorious. Everyone sat outside and food was set-up on the kitchen bar in buffet style. The bar area was across the room set up on my living room desk. It helps to keep food and drink areas separated.

Brunch Menu

Fruit
Watermelon (sliced and quartered)
Strawberries
Cantaloupe or similar melon (thinly sliced)
Grapes
Add your personal favorites
Purchase all on Final Shopping trip. Wash, slice, and put on trays day before event. Cover with plastic wrap or foil.

Meats
Sliced Ham: My favorite is honey baked for maximum flavor, although any spiral ham will work. Purchase up to 3-4 days before event. Separate slices, warm in oven on the morning of event at low temperature for about an hour. Don' t let it dry out.
Bacon: Can cook late in day before or morning of event. Warm in oven on low temperature wrapped in foil.
Sausage: My favorite is Johnsonville Brown Sugar Sausages. The day before, cook in a skillet with water and lid. After tender, drain water and brown in skillet. Warm in oven wrapped in foil on morning of event.
Hint: For optimum oven room, put ham in first and then stack sausages and bacon wrapped in foil on top for last 1/2 hour. Can be served and kept warm in chafing dishes or slow cooker. Also, a good casserole dish with a lid will keep everything warm for quite a while during serving time.

Potatoes
I like to get a 5 lb. bag of small red potatoes. Up to two days before, I wash them well and leave the skin on. Then I cook the potatoes in water until just tender. Don't overcook. Drain and put in refrigerator. The day before the party, quarter the potatoes and brown in skillet with butter and garlic salt. Warm in covered pan in oven on morning of event. Alternatives are packaged au gratin potatoes which are quite good and easy to make. Or you can chop the potatoes and add red and green peppers and onions for more of a hash brown recipe. Also think about using a family favorite.

French Toast
Find good thick bread. Mix egg, milk, and cinnamon in bowl. Dip bread in mixture and place in large skillet coated with vegetable oil. Do several batches until you have the right number of pieces for your guests. After they

are lightly browned put in a covered dish. Refrigerate overnight and warm in oven. Don't forget the softened butter and syrup, which can be warmed on the stove.

Note: For my next brunch I am going to try crepes as one of my choices. They are available at Publix and are very good for being store-made. You can wrap the crepes with ricotta cheese and blueberries with a blueberry glaze for cheese blintzes. Just warm them in the oven. Or you can serve the crepes cold with sliced strawberries and whipped cream.

Scrambled Eggs

This is the only dish in this menu that needs to be made the morning of the party. For 16 people, figure on three dozen eggs – two to three eggs per person. In a large bowl crack the eggs. For very creamy eggs I add heavy cream rather than milk. I like to mix this with a hand mixer to get it very frothy and will result in very fluffy scrambled eggs. In a large skillet slowly melt butter to coat bottom. Right before the butter bubbles, add the egg mixture to about a half inch depth. You may need to do several batches. The secret is to start stirring the eggs immediately and keep stirring until the eggs are shiny. Remove immediately to covered serving dish. Top with salt and pepper. At the last minute you can add grated cheese for some extra flavor and creaminess. Add cheese to skillet right at end of cooking eggs and until just melted.

In addition, I provided some store-bought sliced coffee cakes, Danish, and sweet goodies.

To summarize, the above dishes can all be made the day before except for the scrambled eggs. You will need your oven temperature low and preheated early. You will need oven space for the meats, ham, bacon, and sausage. Best to stack them in the oven. You will also need room to warm the potatoes and French toast. One oven with two shelves will work fine. The only thing for the stovetop are the eggs, and possibly warm syrup.

For the bar you'll need to add to your shopping list:

Orange juice	Tomato juice
Cranberry juice	Celery stalks
Green olives	Limes
Lemons	Strawberries for mimosas?

The tables were decorated with tablecloths topped with sheets of butcher paper. I put glasses with crayons on each table and encouraged each guest to write something on the butcher paper. It made for a fun clean-up!

The centerpieces were lengths of AstroTurf that I purchased at Home Depot. Easter decorations are always fun, and centerpieces were low Easter baskets, filled with Easter grass, candy and little bunnies. The silverware was tied with pink polka dotted ribbon. I had hand painted some wooden Easter eggs with the name of each guest and placed it where I wanted them to sit. Incorporate some Easter decorations in your buffet as well. I painted some small clay flowerpots with the polka dot theme and used them for additional napkins, silverware, and candy. It turned out to be such a nice leisurely afternoon, and everyone had such a "feel-good" time. Including me!

Below are some additional brunch ideas from my talented students:

Sausage and Egg Casserole

2-1/2 cups seasoned croutons
2 cups shredded cheddar cheese
2 pounds pork sausage
8 eggs
1 1/2 cups milk
1 can cream of mushroom soup
1/2 cup evaporated milk

Grease 9x13" pan
Mix eggs and milk together. Set aside. Brown and drain sausage. Layer in pan croutons, 1/2 the cheese, sausage, other half of cheese, beaten eggs and milk mixture. Refrigerate overnight. Mix soup and evaporated milk together and pour the mixture over top. Bake at 300 degrees F. for 1 1/2 hours

APPETIZERS

Call them appetizers, starters, finger foods, hors d'oeuvres, or small bites. By any name, they are a great addition to your party menus. Tasty morsels of an assortment of finger foods are a great way to start off a party or become the star in an all-appetizer cocktail party.

Meatballs are a great staple and are so versatile. Find a favorite from Costco, Sam's, or your favorite grocery store, and keep a bag (or two!) in the freezer. You can warm them in barbecue sauce or chili sauce for an appetizer or put together with your favorite spaghetti sauce for a fast dinner.

Basic Meatballs

If you would like to make the meatballs yourself, below is an easy recipe. Always make a large batch and freeze the extras!

1 lb. lean ground beef
1 egg
2 tbsp. water
1/2 cup breadcrumbs
3 tbsp. minced onion

Preheat oven to 350 degrees F.
Roll into small meatballs and put on cookie sheet.
Bake for 20-25 minutes, turning once.

Lip Smacking Meatballs

2 tbsp. lemon juice
1 small can cranberry jelly
12 oz. bottle of chili sauce (I prefer Hunts)
2 tbsp. brown sugar
36 oz. bag of cooked frozen meatballs

Combine all ingredients in a large saucepan. Heat over low heat until thoroughly mixed and sugar melts.

Serve in slow cooker to keep warm with toothpicks.

For enhanced flavor, refrigerate cooked mixture in refrigerator overnight and reheat on day of event.

Baked Chicken Wings Recipe

1/3 cup flour
2 tbsp. paprika
1 tsp. black pepper
1 teaspoon garlic powder
1 teaspoon salt
3 tbsp. butter
10 chicken wingettes (Wingettes means the tips have been removed)

Preheat oven to 425 degrees F.
Line baking sheet with foil. Dot foil with butter.
In medium bowl combine flour, paprika, garlic powder, salt and pepper. Dab chicken wings with dry paper towel and coat both sides in the flour mixture. Place on baking sheet.
Bake wings for 30 minutes. Turn wings over and bake an additional 15 minutes until crispy.
Serve with favorite dipping sauce and sprinkle with fresh parsley to dress up. Ranch dressing is usually the preferred sauce. Have lots of napkins close by!

Classic Deviled Eggs

I haven't met too many people who don't like deviled eggs! It is one of my favorites to bring to potlucks. I even have a special deviled egg carrier to keep them looking nice after traveling. There is nothing too complicated about making these, even for beginners.

Hard boil eggs and cool. Cut in half lengthwise and put the egg white on plate and yolk in bowl. Mash egg yolk with fork. You can add just mayonnaise, salt and pepper and it's still good. Stuff or pipe mixture into eggs.

If you want to get a little more flavor, add for each 6 eggs:

1/4 cup mayonnaise

1 tsp. white vinegar
1 tsp. yellow mustard
1/8 tsp. salt
Fresh ground pepper
Paprika for garnish

Cheese Balls

Sure, it's old fashioned! It is a traditionally strong well-received goodie! Having a good cheese ball recipe is a great tool in your toolbox of entertaining. You can make it ahead of your party and just pull it out when your guests are coming. Serve with chips, thinly sliced French bread, crackers, sliced vegetables…try what goes best before you serve to your guests.

Basic Cheese Ball

2-8 oz. packages softened cream cheese
1 tsp. seasoned salt
1 small can crushed pineapple, drained
1/4 cup chopped pepper
1/4 cup finely chopped onion
1 cup nuts

Mix all ingredients except nuts. Shape into ball; roll in remaining nuts. Keep refrigerated. This recipe works well with crackers.

Spicy Cheese Ball

8 oz. softened cream cheese
2 cups shredded cheddar cheese
1/4 tsp. onion powder
1/4 tsp. garlic powder
1/4 tsp. cayenne pepper
1/4 cup salsa
1/2 tsp. cumin
2 cups crushed nacho cheese chips

In large bowl, combine cream cheese, shredded cheddar cheese, onion powder, garlic powder, cumin, and salsa. Mix until smooth and well blended. Form mixture into ball and wrap in plastic wrap. Place in refrigerator for at least 2 hours.

Once chilled, remove plastic wrap and roll cheese ball in the crushed nacho chips.

Halloween party idea: Shape ball in shape of pumpkin and place a bell pepper stem on top.

Baked Brie with Caramel and Cranberries
Here's another Cheese idea that looks quite impressive!

1 smaller brie cheese
1/2 cups nuts (pecans good)
1/2 cup dried cranberries (Can substitute or mix blueberries, cherries or plums)
1/4 cup caramel sauce (Same that you would use to make caramel apples)
Ginger crackers (best!) or table crackers

Mix nuts, fruits, and caramel together. Spread over top of the brie and bake for 15 minutes at 350 degrees F.
Serve with crackers.

REGIONAL FAVORITES

The Villages has residents from all over the world who bring their regional favorites for all to share. Here are a few from some of my students:

Candied Kielbasa

3 lbs. package of kielbasa
1 jar chili sauce
2 cans crushed drained pineapple
1/2 cup brown sugar

Cut kielbasa into slices and mix with other ingredients. Put in 9 X 13-inch pan and bake at 350 degrees F. for 1 1/2 hours stirring occasionally. Can be easily transferred to slow cooker for party.

Mexican Roll Ups

10 large flour tortillas
2 pkgs. cream cheese
3 tbsp. mayonnaise
1 small can green chilies
1 small can chopped black olives
1 pkg. taco seasoning
chopped green onions
salsa for dipping

Let tortillas reach room temperature.
Mix all ingredients except tortillas and salsa
Spread mixture thinly over tortillas
Roll tortillas and refrigerate until cheese is firm.
Slice tortillas in 2-inch sections and serve with salsa.

Tortilla Pinwheels

1 pkg. 8 oz. softened cream cheese
1 cup cheddar cheese
1 cup sour cream
1 can (4 1/4) chopped ripe olives
1 4 oz. can chopped green chilies drained
1/2 cup chopped green onions
Garlic powder and salt to taste
5 flour tortillas
Salsa for dipping

Beat cream cheese, cheese, and sour cream until blended. Stir in olives, green chilies, green onions, and seasonings.

Spread over tortillas and roll up tightly. Wrap each in plastic twisting ends to seal. Refrigerate for several hours.

Unwrap. Cut into 1/2-to-3/4-inch slices. Serve with salsa.

Texas Caviar

<u>Drain and mix together:</u>
15.5 oz. can black eyed peas
15.5 oz. can pimento beans
small jar chopped pimentos
15 oz. can white shoe peg corn
1 small, chopped onion
1 chopped green pepper
<u>Marinade</u>:
1 tsp. salt
1/2 tsp. pepper
1 tbsp. water
1/4 cup oil
3/4 cup cider vinegar
3/4 to 1 cup sugar

Heat marinade to boiling. Pour over other ingredients. Let mixture sit for 2 hours or more in the refrigerator. Drain most of the marinade off before serving.

Serve with lime Dorito chips or scoop Fritos.

Sausage Cups

1 lb. hot sausage
16 oz pkg. Won ton wrappers
1 cup shredded Monterey Jack Cheese
1 cup shredded Cheddar cheese
1/2 cup ranch dressing

Preheat oven to 350 degrees F.

Crumble sausage into medium skillet. Cook over medium heat until lightly browned, stirring occasionally. Drain.

Spray mini muffin tins and insert won ton wrappers to form a small cup.

Bake 5 minutes in preheated oven. Allow wrappers to cool.

Mix sausage, cheeses and ranch dressing together. Fill won ton wrapper cups. Bake 10-12 minutes until bubbly.

Puffy Pancakes

4 servings (multiply for number of guests)

6 eggs
1 cup all-purpose flour
1 cup milk
1/2 cup sugar
1/4 cup frozen orange juice concentrate
1 stick plus 1 tbsp. butter

Garnish with lemon wedges, powdered sugar, and fresh berries, sweetened.

Combine eggs, flour, milk, sugar and orange juice in blender or food processor and mix well. Add 1 tbsp. butter and blend in thoroughly.

Add 1 tbsp. butter to each of four oval or round baking dishes (ramekins are perfect). Heat dishes in oven until butter is melted but not browned.

Divide batter evenly among dishes. Bake until puffed and golden, about 20 minutes.

Serve immediately with lemon wedges, powdered sugar and fresh berries.

Cheesy Hash Brown Bake

1 pkg. (30 oz.) frozen shredded hash brown potatoes (thawed)
2 cans (10 1/2 oz.) condensed cream of potato soup undiluted
2 cups sour cream
2 cups shredded Cheddar cheese
1 cup Parmesan cheese

In bowl combine the hash browns, soup, sour cream, 1 3/4 cups Cheddar cheese, and Parmesan cheese. Transfer to a greased 3-quart baking dish.

Sprinkle with remaining Cheddar cheese.

Bake uncovered at 350 degrees F. for 40-45 minutes or until bubbly or cheese is melted. Let stand 5 minutes before serving.

DIPS

Dips are a great staple. Have several recipes that you find easy to put together and that are well received. If you choose to go with a store-bought dip, make sure you do a taste test. Serve with chips, crackers, veggie sticks of carrots, celery, or pepper, or thinly sliced crusty bread. They are also easy to make ahead!

Spinach Artichoke Dip

4 oz. Alouette Garlic and Herb Spreadable cheese
4 cloves garlic
1/2 cup chopped scallions (green onion is fine)
4 tbsp. butter
2 10 oz. pkg. chopped frozen spinach, cooked and drained
1 tsp. salt
2 8oz. cans artichoke hearts drained
1/2 tsp. pepper
1/4 cup grated parmesan cheese
2 cups heavy cream

Sauté scallions and chopped garlic in butter. Add spinach and artichokes on low heat. Add cream, alouette cheese, salt, and pepper. Simmer until blended. Remove from heat and fold in Parmesan cheese.

Hot Artichoke Dip

1-14 oz. can (not jar) artichoke hearts, drained and chopped fine
1-8 oz. pkg. cream cheese (soften in microwave for easy stirring)
1 c. freshly grated Parmesan cheese
1/2 cup real mayonnaise
1/2 tsp. each salt, oregano, and garlic powder
1/4 tsp. garlic salt

Mix all ingredients. Can be refrigerated at this point and baked later. When ready to bake, place in baking dish about 7 x 11. I like a large ovenproof au gratin dish. Bake covered at 350 degrees for 30 minutes. Uncover and continue baking until top is bubbly and a soft golden brown. Recipe can be doubled and will fill a 9 X 13 dish. Great traveler dish!

Buffalo Chicken Dip

2-10 oz. cans chunk chicken, drained
2-8 oz. packages cream cheese, softened
1 cup Ranch dressing
1/2 cup red hot pepper sauce
1-1/2 cups shredded cheddar cheese

Heat chicken and hot sauce in skillet over medium heat. Stir in cream cheese and ranch dressing. Cook until well blended and warm. Mix in half of Cheddar cheese and transfer to slow cooker. Sprinkle remaining cheese over top. Cook on low setting until hot and bubbly.

The following two recipes contain Rotel (brand name), which is diced tomatoes and green chiles mixed. Great to buy several cans and keep in your pantry for those last minutes parties!

Rotel Sausage Dip

1 pound pork sausage
2 8 oz. packages softened cream cheese
2 10 oz. cans diced tomatoes and green chiles (like Rotel), well drained
1/2 tsp. garlic powder
pinch of salt

Brown sausage in a skillet until cooked through and drain fat. Add cooked sausage, cream cheese, diced tomatoes and green chilies, garlic and salt to a crock pot and heat until bubbly, stirring occasionally. Easy recipe to change up adding green onions, or Parmesan cheese.

Velveeta Spicy Cheeseburger Dip

1 lb. (16 oz.) Velveeta, cut into 1/2-inch cubes
1 can (10 oz.) Rotel Diced tomatoes and green chilies, undrained
1 cup shredded low-moisture part-skim mozzarella cheese

1/2 lb. ground beef, cooked, drained
4 green onions, sliced

Mix all ingredients except onions in a microwaveable bowl. Microwave on high 5 minutes or until Velveeta is melted, stirring after 3 minutes. Stir in onions. Perfect to then put in slow cooker to keep warm.

Million Dollar Dip

1 1/2 cup mayonnaise
1 cup shredded Cheddar Cheese
4 chopped green onions
1/2 cup really bacon bits
1/2 cup slivered almonds
1 tsp. garlic, minced

In a large bowl, add the mayonnaise, cheddar cheese, green onions, bacon bits, almonds, and garlic. Use a spatula to thoroughly mix.

CHEESE

The MAGIC ingredient that is always a crowd pleaser! It can be used in so many successful recipes and I can't think of anything as versatile or valuable in party planning.

Parmesan Cheese Straws

1 egg
1 sheet thawed frozen puff pastry
1/2 cup grated Parmesan cheese
1/2 tsp. kosher salt
1/2 tsp. paprika
1/4 tsp. cayenne
Flour to roll pastry
1 tbsp. water

Beat one egg with 1 tablespoon water. Roll out 1 sheet thawed frozen puff pastry into a 12-inch square on floured surface. Brush with beaten egg and sprinkle with 1/2 cup grated Parmesan, 1/2 teaspoon each kosher salt and paprika, and 1/4 teaspoon cayenne.

Cut into 24 strips 1/2 inch thick.

Bake at 375 degrees F. until golden for 15 minutes

Chile Cheese Straws

Make Cheese straws above replacing Parmesan with shredded Cheddar cheese. Use smoked paprika and sprinkle dough with 1 teaspoon chili powder.

Prosciutto-Parmesan Palmiers

1 sheet thawed frozen puff pastry
1/4 cup grated Parmesan cheese
1 oz. sliced Prosciutto.
Roll out 1 sheet of frozen puff pastry into a 12-inch square on a floured surface. Cut in half; cover each half with 1/4 cup grated Parmesan cheese and

1 oz. Prosciutto. Roll the short sides of each rectangle toward the center so the two ends meet in the middle. Gently press together and freeze until firm. Trim the ends and slice each log 1/4 inch thick.

Bake at 400 degrees F. until golden; 12 to 15 minutes.

Sausage Cheddar Bites

Summer sausage sliced into 1/4-inch rounds
Grated cheddar cheese
Butter crackers

Top 1/4-inch-thick rounds of summer sausage with sliced cheddar. Bake at 375 degrees F. until the cheese melts (3-5 minutes).

Sandwich between butter crackers

Gorgonzola Cheese Dip

3/4 cup Sour cream
1/2 cup crumbled Gorgonzola
1 tbsp. milk
Salt
Cayenne pepper
Assorted cut vegetables for dip

Combine all ingredients and serve with vegetables.

Caraway-Havarti Beer Cheese

1/2 stick butter
1/4 cup flour
1 cup heavy cream
1 cup beer
1 tbsp. Dijon mustard
1/2 tsp. kosher salt
hot sauce to taste
2 cups shredded Caraway Havarti Cheese

Melt 1/2 cup stick butter over medium heat. Stir in 1/4 cup flour and cook, stirring 2 minutes. Add one cup each heavy cream and beer, 1 tablespoon Dijon mustard and 1/2 teaspoon each kosher salt and hot sauce. Simmer 5 minutes. Stir in 2 cups shredded Caraway Havarti until melted. Serve with chips. Perfect for an Oktoberfest party!

Spanakopita Tartlets

10 oz. pkg. frozen spinach
1/2 cup crumbled feta cheese
2 tbsp. chopped scallions
2 tbsp. chopped dill
30 frozen mini phyllo shells

Cook frozen spinach as directed and drain. Stir in 1/2 cup crumbled feta and 2 tablespoons each chopped scallions and dill. Fill 30 frozen mini phyllo shells with mixture.

Bake at 400 degrees F. until set about 15 minutes.
Cool slightly before serving.

Cheese Puffs

1 stick butter
1/2 cup milk
1/2 cup water
1/4 tsp. kosher salt
1/4 tsp. cayenne pepper
1 cup flour
4 eggs
1 cup grated Gruyere cheese

Bring butter, water, milk salt and cayenne to a simmer in a saucepan. Stir in flour until a ball forms. Transfer to a bowl and with a mixer beat in eggs one at a time. Add Gruyere.

Pipe or drop by 1-inch balls on baking sheet covered with parchment paper. Bake at 400 degrees F. until puffed, about 25 minutes.

SALADS

Salads are a great choice to bring to a potluck or to have on your own buffet. Below are some of the favorites and "go to" recipes from my creative students.

Fruit Salad

2 cans chunk pineapple
2 1/2 cans sliced pears
1 large jar maraschino cherries (no stems or pits)
2 small cans mandarin oranges
4 bananas
1 pkg. REGULAR vanilla pudding mix (not instant —use cook and serve)

Save cherry juice and one can of pineapple juice in separate cups. Drain the rest of the fruit and place in a bowl. Pour pudding mix into small saucepan. Add 1 cup of juice (cherry plus needed pineapple to equal one cup).

Stir and cook until thick. Set aside to cool. Pour cooled pudding mixture over the bowl of drained fruit. Refrigerate. Just before serving add bananas. This salad will keep for a few days in refrigerator and can be made a day ahead of the event. The red cherries are very festive for the holidays.

Asian Salad

Dressing-Make ahead and let sit for at least an hour
2/3 cup oil
1/3 cup apple cider vinegar
1/2 to 2/3 cup sugar
2 pkg. beef flavoring from beef flavored Ramen noodles
Salad
12 oz. bag cole slaw
1/4 to 1/2 bag broccoli slaw
1 cup roasted sunflower seeds
2 bunches chopped green onions
1 cup slivered almonds
2 pkg. beef ramen noodles broken apart

Put noodles in large zip lock bag, seal and break apart the noodles. Add to the bag the sunflower seeds and almonds and set aside until serving. Right before serving top with salad dressing and toss together.

Granny's Ambrosia Salad

8 oz. Cool Whip
1/2 cup sour cream
11 oz. mandarin oranges drained
20 oz. crushed pineapple drained
10 oz. maraschino cherries drained
1 cup shredded coconut
2 cups marshmallows

Fold together Cool Whip and sour cream in a large mixing bowl until completely mixed.

Stir in the drained mandarins and pineapple, followed by coconut and marshmallows

Drain and press the cherries between 2 sheets of paper towel, then carefully stir into the ambrosia said to prevent bruising. Refrigerate at least 2 hours before serving.

Supreme Pasta Salad

1 package (16 oz.) Penne, Rotini, or bow tie pasta
5 cups assorted vegetables (broccoli florets, bell pepper, cherry tomato)
1 bottle (8 oz.) Italian dressing
McCormick Salad Supreme Seasoning to taste.

Cook pasta as directed. Rinse under cold water; drain

Place pasta and veggies in bowl. Add dressing and seasoning. Toss gently to coat. Cover.

Refrigerate at least 4 hours. Toss before serving.

Broccoli Salad

8 oz. bacon
salt
5 cups small broccoli florets
1 cup mayonnaise
1 tbsp. apple cider vinegar
1/3 cup chopped onion
3/4 cup raisins
1/2 cup sunflower kernels
chopped green olives

Cut bacon into small pieces and cook over medium heat until just crisp; drain on paper towels. Bring a large saucepan of salted water to a boil. Add the broccoli and blanch until bright green and slightly softened, about 3 minutes. Drain well, run under cold water to stop the cooking, and drain again.

In a mixing bowl, combine the mayonnaise, vinegar, onion, and raisins. Add the broccoli and toss and coat with dressing. Refrigerate for one hour.

Just before serving, fold in the sunflower kernels and bacon pieces. Serve immediately.

When we catered weddings, we always would offer several salads for guests. Here are 3 of my favorites:

Cooper's Catering Fruit Salad

Watermelon cut into bite sized chunks
grapes
cut strawberries
Cantaloupe cup into bite sized chunks
Blueberries
Raspberries

No dressing. Just pure fruit goodness. Mix and let the flavors come together overnight. Beautifully served in a hollowed-out watermelon cut with a handle like a watermelon basket.

Cooper's Catering Famous Easy Potato Salad

5 lbs. potatoes (can use russet, red, or Yukon gold)
6 stalks celery chopped
8 eggs
1 red apple (fuji is good)
Mayonnaise
Salt and pepper to taste

Cook potatoes until tender. Do not overcook. Drain and cool. Cook eggs and hard boil. Drain and cool. Chop celery and apple (leave red skin on) Mix all together with mayonnaise and salt and pepper. Chill. The apple adds a surprise sweetness.

Cooper's Catering Favorite Italian Pasta Salad

16 oz. pasta (bowtie, small penne, macaroni)
1 can pitted medium Black olives
3 fresh tomatoes
1/2 cup grated parmesan cheese
1 cucumber chopped into bite sized pieces
1 green onion sliced
2 stalks sliced celery
1/2 red bell pepper sliced thin
1 pkg. Good Seasons Italian Salad dressing mixed with oil and vinegar according to directions.

Cook pasta, drain, and cool. Mix other ingredients together with pasta and top with Italian Dressing Chill overnight. Can add canned mushrooms, artichoke hearts, or your personal favorite vegetable.

MAIN DISHES

You can use these main dishes for a potluck or buffet. You can also adapt them to dinner parties. When having a formal dinner party, you can choose to have a Buffet set up where your guests serve themselves, or you can serve it family-style. Serving family style is a little more intimate and gives the party more of a formal feel. However, for larger dinner parties, a buffet is a better way to go.

THE STAR ATTRACTION

For a buffet, and even more so for a dinner party, you should have a main attraction. A main dish that you build the rest of your menu around. It could be a roasted Tenderloin of Beef, a whole baked salmon, or a large Virginia Ham, which are all best suited for a smaller Dinner Party. If you are planning a large buffet or Dinner Party, consider a casserole or a large pasta dish. Casseroles can usually be put together the day before and then just warmed up in the Oven, freeing you up to enjoy your party!

Easy Chicken Breasts

The recipe below is only for 4 people. Multiply ingredients to reflect how many servings you need. Easy, in that you can put it together, stick it in the refrigerator, and then throw it in the oven.

4 boneless chicken breast halves
1 cup mayonnaise
1/2 cup fresh grated or shredded parmesan
1 1/2 tsp. seasoning salt
1/2 tsp. black pepper
1 tsp. garlic powder

Preheat oven to 375 degrees F. Mix mayonnaise, cheese, seasonings. Spread and cover each chicken piece with mixture. Place on baking dish. Putting foil down first will make it easier to clean up.
Bake for 45 minutes.

Chicken Marsala

This is a recipe for 4 people. Multiply as needed.

1 tsp. minced garlic
1 tsp. Marjoram leaves
1 tsp. basil leaves
1/4 cup flour
1 tsp. salt
1/4 black pepper
1 lb. thinly sliced boneless skinless chicken breasts
3 tbsp. butter, divided
2 tbsp. olive oil
1 8 oz. pkg. sliced mushrooms
3/4 cup chicken stock or broth
1/2 cup dry Marsala wine

Mix flour, minced garlic, marjoram, salt, and pepper in a shallow dish. Reserve 1 tablespoon flour mixture. Coat chicken with remaining flour mixture.

Heat 2 tablespoons of the butter and oil in large nonstick skillet on medium high heat. Cook chicken in batches 3 minutes each side or until golden brown. Remove from skillet and keep warm. Add mushrooms to skillet. Cook and stir 5 minutes or until tender.

Mix stock and reserved flour mixture. Add to skillet with wine. Bring to a boil, stirring to release browned bits in bottom of skillet. Stir in remaining 1 tablespoon butter and basil. Cook 2 minutes or until sauce is slightly thickened. If sauce is too thick, add more Marsala to thin.

Mozzarella Stuffed Meatloaf

1-1/2 pounds lean ground beef
1 cup breadcrumbs
1 tsp. dried basil
1 tsp. dried oregano
1 tsp. dried parsley
1 tsp. salt
1/2 tsp. black pepper

1/2 cup milk
2 tbsp. Worcestershire sauce
8 oz. fresh mozzarella cheese sliced

Glaze
1 cup ketchup 1/4 cup brown sugar lightly packed
1 tbsp. Worcestershire sauce
1 tbsp. red wine vinegar
2 crushed cloves garlic
1/8 tsp. salt

Preheat oven to 350 Degrees F. Lightly grease a 9x13 pan with cooking spray. I like to use a glass one.

In large mixing bowl combine ground beef, breadcrumbs, basil, oregano, parsley, salt, pepper, milk, and Worcestershire sauce. Knead until combined.

Divide meat in half. Shape one half into the bottom half of the loaf and place in prepared pan. Place mozzarella cheese down the center. Shape remaining half of meat as the top half and place on top of the mozzarella cheese. Seal the edges all the way around.

In small mixing bowl mix together all the items in the Glaze. Pour half of the mixture over the meatloaf. Reserve the other half for later.

Bake for 45 minutes, remove from oven and pour the remaining glaze over the loaf. Increase oven temperature to 400 degrees F. and bake for 15 more minutes.

Let rest about 10 minutes before serving.

Chicken and Jack Cheese Quesadillas

These would work as a main course, or you can cut them with a pizza cutter for appetizers.
3 cups chicken broth or water
1/2 tsp. salt
3 skinless, boneless chicken breast halves

4 large flour tortillas; 10-12 inches in diameter
2 cups shredded Monterey Jack Cheese
1/2 cup sour cream
4 tbsp. store bought fresh tomato salsa, plus 1/2 cup for serving

In a deep pan or saucepan bring broth or water to a simmer over medium high heat. Add chicken breast halves and simmer until just opaque, about 10-12 minutes. This will make them very tender. Remove from heat and let chicken cool in the liquid. Lift out and shred into bite sized pieces. You should have about 2 cups of shredded chicken.

Pour a little cooking oil in a large skillet or use nonstick cooking spray. When hot, place tortilla in pan and sprinkle with one fourth of the shredded cheese. Top with one fourth of the shredded chicken and one tablespoon of the salsa.

Fold the tortilla in half, pressing down with a spatula. Cook until lightly browned on one side and then turn over and brown the other side. Repeat to make 4 tortillas in all.

Can be kept warm in the oven until serving.

Chow Mein Hamburger Casserole

Brown in skillet:
2 lbs. hamburger meat
1 1/2 cup chopped celery
2 chopped onions
1/2 tsp. salt
Add:
1 cup raw rice
2 cups water
4 tbsp. soy sauce
1 can cream of chicken soup
1 can cream of mushroom soup
1 can bean sprouts

Cover and bake in oven for 1 hour at 325 degrees F.

Easy Tomato Bean Bake

Cooking spray
28 oz. can Bush's Original (or vegetarian) Baked Beans
14.5 oz. can Bush's low sodium black beans, drained
14.5 oz. can Hunts fire roasted diced tomatoes (not drained)
1 1/2 cups chopped onion
1/4 cup molasses
1/2 tsp. Worcestershire sauce
If not vegetarian add 4 slices raw bacon. If vegetarian but not dairy free, 1/4 cup parmesan cheese. If vegetarian, 1 tbsp. paprika

Preheat oven to 425 degrees F. Coat a 2.5- or 3-quart baking dish with cooking spray

In large mixing bowl, dump everything except bacon (or cheese and paprika). Mix.

Transfer bean mixture to baking dish. If using bacon, lay slices across top of beans. If adding Parmesan cheese or paprika, add after baking.

Bake uncovered 25-30 minutes or until bacon is browned and sauce bubbles around edges.

Let stand 5 minutes before serving. Can be made a day ahead.

POTATOES

Potatoes are under-appreciated in their party usefulness. I had one student who chose to honor the lowly potato with a party celebrating ONLY the potato on National Potato Day. Every dish had potato in the ingredients, yet she was able to create a varied and interesting menu. Who was the star in her decorations? Of course, Mr. Potato Head!

Baked Yukon Gold Potatoes

Scrub potatoes. Roll in olive oil. Roll in kosher salt. Bake in casserole for 2 hours at 325 degrees F. They will be crispy on the outside. Use Yukon potatoes only. Easy perfect companion for many main courses.

Sour Cream Mashed Potatoes

Large box of instant mashed potatoes (enough for 18 servings)
16 oz. softened cream cheese
2 cup sour cream
2 tsp. garlic salt
1 tsp. garlic powder
2 tsp. fresh chives
2 tbsp. butter

Prepare 18 servings of instant mashed potatoes in a large Dutch oven or large pot.

Stir in cream cheese, sour cream, garlic salt, garlic powder and chives into the hot potatoes. Adjust to taste with seasonings.

Potatoes can be refrigerated and baked later. Bake covered to start at 350-375 degrees F. Baking temperature and time will vary if potatoes are refrigerated.

Remove cover and let top become golden brown. Baking time can take up to an hour, but these are so good and go with so many different proteins - beef, fish, pork, ham.

Mashed Potato Puffs

These are great for a buffet style dinner party. Makes 12-24 puffs, depending on size.

Cooking spray or butter
2 cups cooked mashed potatoes
3 large eggs, beaten
Sour cream for serving
1 cup grated cheese (parmesan or Gruyere, divided)
1/4 cup minced chives
1/4 cup cooked bacon or ham (optional)
kosher salt and pepper to taste

Arrange rack in middle of oven and heat to 400 degrees F. Lightly coat the cups of a mini-muffin tin with cooking spray or butter.

Place mashed potatoes, eggs, 3/4 cup cheese, chives, and bacon or ham in large bowl and stir to combine. Season with salt and pepper.

Fill each muffin cup with mashed potato mixture. Sprinkle top with remaining 1/4 cup cheese.

Bake until potatoes are browned on top, and heated through, about 20 minutes. Let cool about 5 minutes before gently removing them from the pan. Serve immediately with dollops of sour cream.

Leftovers can be stored in an airtight container in the refrigerator for up to 3 days. To reheat and re-crisp, arrange the puffs on a baking sheet.

Bake at 400 degrees F for about 15 minutes.

Cheesy Hash Brown Bake

Thaw 1 pkg (30 oz.) frozen shredded hash browns
2 cans condensed Cream of Potato sour undiluted
2 cup sour cream
2 cups shredded cheddar cheese (divided)

1 cup grated parmesan cheese

In bowl, combine the potatoes, soup, sour cream, 1-3/4 cups cheddar cheese and the Parmesan Cheese.

Transfer to greased 3-quart baking dish. Sprinkle with remaining Cheddar cheese. Bake uncovered at 350 degrees F for 40-45 minutes or until bubbly and cheese is melted.

Let stand 5 minutes before serving.

DESSERTS

Desserts are optional and dependent upon what kind of party you are having. Or you might be having a party that is JUST desserts. In Europe, it is customary to have a good cheese and fruit for dessert. It is a very nice end to a good meal.

Another easy fix is a scoop of quality ice cream, sherbet, or gelato, with some wonderful cookies. Below are some ideas. Try to find some favorites that are easy to make ahead.

Refrigerator Cookies

1 cup shortening
1 cup white sugar
2 eggs
1 1/2 tsp. vanilla extract
3 cups all-purpose flour
1 tsp. salt
1/2 tsp. baking soda
1/3 cup colored sugar for decoration

Mix shortening, sugar, eggs, and vanilla together in large bowl. Stir flour, salt, and baking soda together in a separate bowl. Blend dry ingredients in with the shortening mixture. Mix thoroughly by hand. Divide dough into 3 parts. Shape into cylinders, 1-1/2 inches in diameter and about 7 inches long. Roll in colored sugar or finely chopped nuts. Chill for several hours or overnight.

Heat oven to 400 degrees F. Cut into 1/4-inch slices and place on greased cookie sheets. Bake for 8-10 minutes. Cool. Will freeze well for several months! Always double the recipe and have cookies ready to cook for any occasion.

Cookie Fruit Tart

1/2 of a 20 oz. roll refrigerated sugar cookie dough
4 oz. light cream cheese such as Neufchatel
1/4 cup sour cream
2 tsp. sugar
2-1/2 cups fruit such as sliced strawberries and peaches, blueberries, raspberry

Heat oven to 350 degrees F.

With lightly floured fingers, pat cookie dough in to a 9-inch circle on uncreased cookie sheet.

Bake 12-14 minutes until golden. Cool 5 minutes.

Loosen cookie with a spatula, then slide onto rack to cool completely.
Mix cream cheese, sour cream, and sugar in a small bowl with a wooden spoon until blended.
Place cookie on serving plate. Spread cream cheese mixture to within 1/2 inch of edge. Arrange fruit on top. Serve or refrigerate up to 2 hours. To serve, cut in wedges.

Serves 8. Great for dessert or brunch.

Chocolate Lasagna

1 package regular Oreo cookies (not double stuff) about 36 cookies
6 tbsp. melted butter
8 oz. package softened cream cheese
1/4 cup granulated sugar
2 tbsp. cold milk
12 oz. tub Cool whip, divided
1-1/2 cups mini chocolate chips
2 pkgs. (3.9 oz each) Chocolate instant pudding
3-1/4 cups cold milk

Begin by crushing cookies either in food processor or crushed with rolling pin in plastic bag until fine crumbs. Transfer Oreo crumbs to large bowl.

Stir in 6 tablespoons melted butter and use fork to incorporate the butter into cookie crumbs.

Transfer to 9x13 baking dish. Press crumbs into bottom of pan. Place the pan in the refrigerator.

Mix the cream cheese until light and fluffy Add in 2 tablespoons milk and sugar and mix well.

Stir in 1-1/4 cups Cool Whip. Spread this mixture over crust.

Combine chocolate instant pudding with 3-1/4 cups cold milk. Whisk for several minutes until pudding starts to thicken. Use a spatula to spread the mixture over the previous cream cheese layer.
Allow dessert to rest for about 5 minutes while it thickens further.

Spread remaining Cool Whip over the top. Sprinkle mini chocolate chips evenly over the top. Place in freezer for 1 hour, or the refrigerator for 4 hours before serving.

Raw Apple Cake

2 cups flour
2 cups sugar
4 cups chopped, skinless apples
4 tsp. cinnamon
1 1/2 tsp. baking soda
1 1/2 tsp. salt
2 eggs
1 cup shortening/ canola oil
1 cup chopped pecans
2 tsp. vanilla

Preheat oven to 350 degrees F. Bring all ingredients to room temperature.

Mix dry ingredients, then wet ingredients, then add apples and nuts in a large mixing bowl.

Place mixed ingredients into greased Bundt pan. Bake for 1 hour. Let cool for about 20 minutes before turning pan over and cooling for another 15 -20 minutes.

Optional topping: Bring 1 stick butter, 4 tablespoons cream/ milk, 1 cup brown sugar to boil. Remove from heat and stir in chopped pecans. Pour over completely cooled cake. Cake can be served warm with vanilla ice cream for a new favorite.

Can also be great for brunch!

Coffee Cake

1 box yellow cake mix
1 small carton sour cream
3/4 cup hot water
4 eggs
1/4 cup Crisco oil
1 pkg. vanilla instant pudding

Mix all above ingredients together. In separate bowl mix:

1/2 cup sugar
2 tsp. cinnamon
1/2 cup chopped nuts

Grease Bundt cake pan. Alternate the sugar mixture with the cake mixture.

Bake at 350 degrees for 35-45 minutes. Let cake cool in pan before removing. Drizzle thin icing over cake.

A good basic cake which can be tasty anytime of the day Breakfast, brunch, dessert with fruit on top?

Million Dollar Pound Cake

4 cups sifted flour
1 pound salted softened butter (4 sticks)
1 tbsp. pure vanilla extract
1 tsp. almond extract
3 cups granulated sugar
6 large eggs
3/4 cup whole milk or buttermilk

Preheat oven to 300 degrees F. Butter and flour an angel food/ tube pan with a removable bottom. Set aside. In bowl of stand mixer using the whisk attachment combine the butter, vanilla, and almond extract. Whip for 5 minutes on medium high.

Switch to paddle attachment. Add the sugar gradually beating on medium until light yellow in color around 5 minutes.

Add the eggs one at a time beating well after each addition. Scrape sides of the bowl as needed.

Lower the speed of the mixer and add the flour alternately with the milk, beginning and ending with flour. Stop and scrape the sides of the bowl occasionally.

After all has been added, beat for 1-2 minutes until the flour has incorporated. Spread evenly into pan and bounce on counter to level.

Bake for 1 hour 30-45 minutes or until toothpick comes back clean. Cool for 15 minutes and remove the outer ring.

This cake can be made in a tube pan without a removable bottom.

Cathy's Holiday Bars

2 cups whole cranberries
2 cups sugar
4 eggs
2 cups flour
1 cup nuts (pecans good)
1-1/2 tsp. almond extract
1 1/2 cups melted butter (3 sticks)

Beat eggs, add sugar, flour, almond extract, and melted butter. Add the nuts, then gently fold in cranberries. Pour into an 11 X 15 greased cookie sheet.

Bake at 350 degrees F for 30 minutes.
Make glaze of 1 cup powdered sugar, 1/2 teaspoon almond extract and milk. Drizzle over bars once they are cooled.

Pumpkin Gingerbread Trifle

2-14 oz. pkgs. gingerbread mix
5.1 oz. box cook and serve vanilla pudding mix
30 oz. can pumpkin pie filling
1/2 cup packed brown sugar
1/3 tsp. ground cardamom or cinnamon
12 oz. container frozen whipped topping
1/2 cup gingersnaps (optional)

Bake the gingerbread according to the package directions; cool completely. Prepare the pudding and set aside to cool. Stir the pumpkin pie filling, sugar, and cardamom into the pudding. Crumble 1 batch of gingerbread into the bottom of a large pretty (preferably clear glass) bowl. Pour 1/2 of the pudding mixture over the gingerbread, then add a layer of whipped topping. Repeat with the remaining gingerbread, pudding, and whipped topping. Sprinkle the top with crushed gingersnaps. Refrigerate overnight.

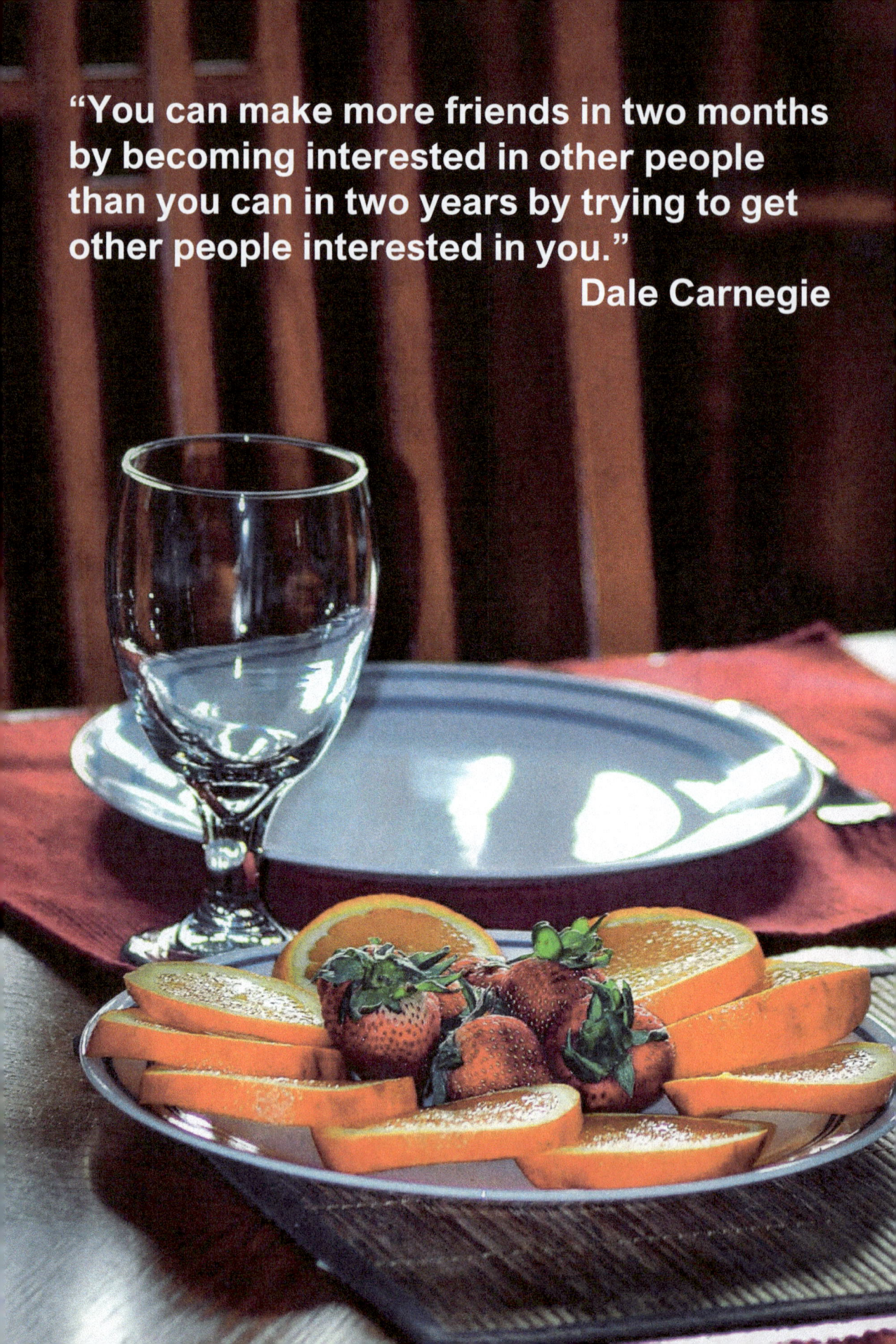

Chapter 8
Entertaining is Magical

Life is to be celebrated! I love sharing this information with you especially since the pandemic has taught us how important and precious relationships are and how special time spent together is for happiness.

It is my wish that this book will be helpful to you in putting together a useful plan for having wonderful parties. A wonderful host and memorable event do not require a Master Chef, but it does require a masterful party planner.

I hope this book becomes a reference for you and that you refer to it often for your party planning and entertaining. The best parties are those that you can enjoy yourself. The systems that I have laid out for you have been successfully used over many years and are invaluable in keeping you organized and on track. Your preparation and lists will keep you in control of any doubts or butterflies. Your confidence will soar with each successful party as your invitation becomes THAT one which everyone wants to receive. I hope your parties will be those that people talk about for years to come.

Most importantly, the lesson learned is to have fun, gather together with loved ones, make new friends, and reunite with your family. Make it joyful, make it special, and cherish making memories together with extreme laughter!

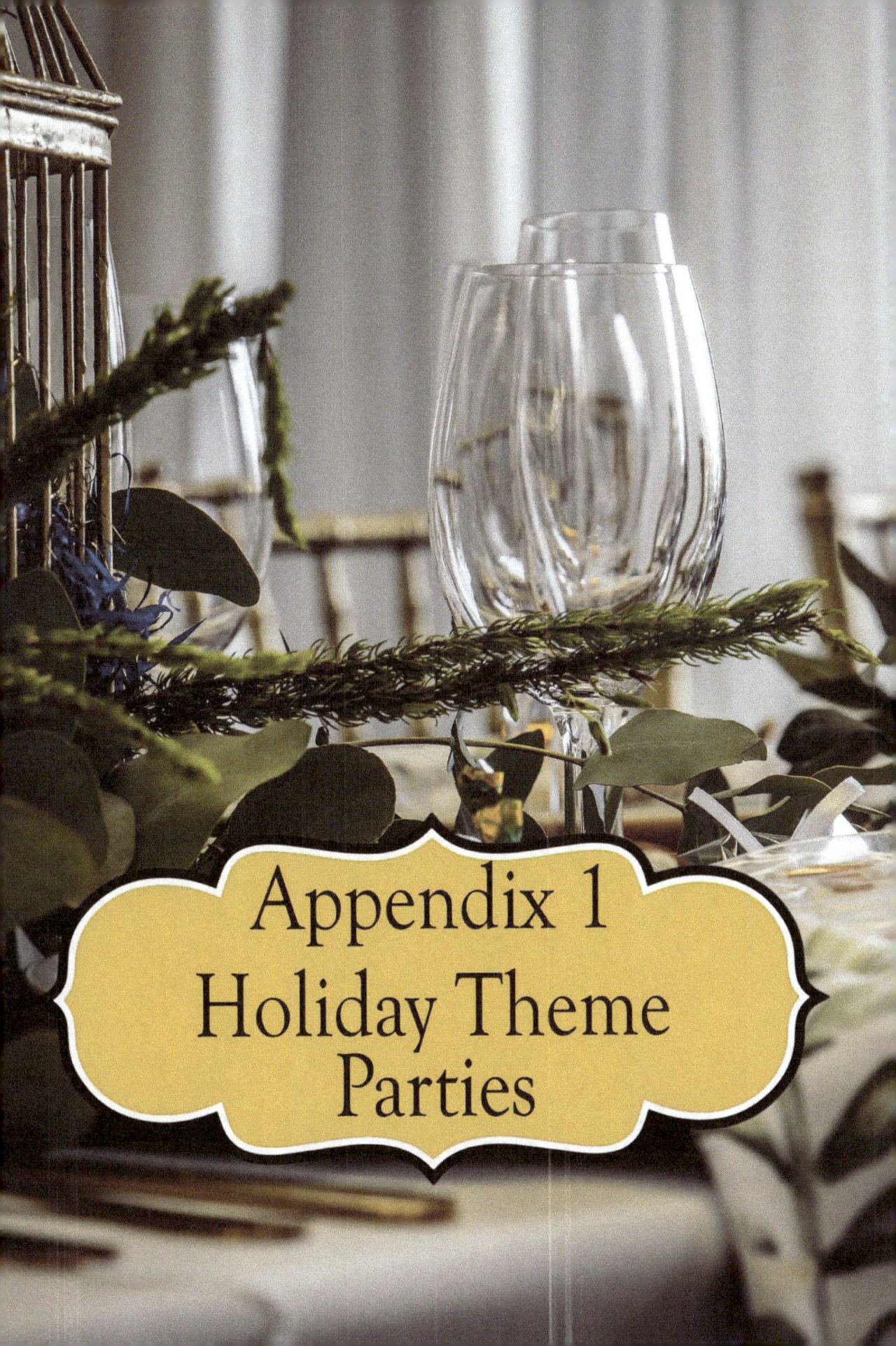
Appendix 1
Holiday Theme Parties

List of Holiday Theme Parties

Below are some holiday theme party suggestions that can easily be developed, elevated, and even mixed together. Most parties lend themselves to a potluck, cocktail, or buffet type of party. You could plan an Appetizer-Only Potluck, or a Dessert-Only Potluck, as an easy menu.

Mr. and Mrs. Claus Dress-Up Party - Rent a photo booth and plan Christmas card sharing.

Pet-mas Party—Dogs are part of our families! Everyone brings their precious fur balls dressed in their holiday finest. Remember treats for your furry friends: Supply plastic bags for bathroom trips, water bowls, and a photo booth. Owner and fur ball dressed alike? Have prizes for the best costumes.

Christmas Shopping Soup-to-Nuts Party - Have a gift wrap station set up for wrapping gifts. Have a supply of scissors, paper, ribbons, tape, gift tags, and more with a large worktable.

Christmas Carol Karaoke Party - Have a supply of words to favorite Christmas songs and a playlist so that everyone can follow along. Serve hot chocolate, hot toddies, and dessert.

Christmas Angel Party - Make everyone an angel that comes to your party. You supply the wings and halos which are available on Amazon. This is a great party to coordinate for a "Party with a Purpose." Absolutely have a photo booth.

Christmas Movie Party – What if everyone had to take a shot of liquid every time "Merry Christmas" was mentioned? Have designated drivers available, depending on the movie.

Ladies Only Wine Night and Beauty Gift Exchange – This one is always fun and well attended. Gifts could include feminine luxury items like body lotion, bubble bath, a gift certificate for a mani-pedi or a massage.

Men Only Football and Bourbon Christmas Celebration – This one speaks for itself and could involve some betting or fun games. Have a supply of chips, popcorn, nuts, and finger foods.

Christmas High Tea and Crafting Afternoon with the Ladies - Have projects, supplies, and instructions available. This one could include a cookie exchange.

Feliz Navidad Party - Have Mexican food and Margaritas! A piñata with Christmas gifts. Could be a focal point. Serve Mexican food which is particularly easy to prepare and serve.

Christmas Dessert Party- Schedule a party for after dinner with many different kinds of dessert and sweets. Pair with great coffee, coffee drinks, and liquors.

Pancakes and Pajamas Christmas Party – This is especially fun if your party is for neighbors only.

Christmas Brunch Party -An easy party to develop, this could include outside seating in good weather, and is surprisingly easy to execute and elevate.

Mad-For-Plaid Christmas Party - Incorporate your decorations with a plaid theme. All guests should be asked to wear plaid. Easy to mix with a potluck or cocktail party

Giving Back Christmas Party – This one always contributes to that warm and fuzzy Christmas feeling. Have guests bring children's Christmas gifts to donate, or food for a local food bank—you choose your favorite. Try to find a big sleigh where gifts can be dropped. Either have each gift specified as to age group, if it is wrapped, or supply a gift wrap station and separate them at that point. Providing information about the cause where you are donating is always appreciated and emailing a video of the delivery (if possible) is always a very nice thank you to the giver.

The following parties could work the week BETWEEN Christmas and New Year's or even the week AFTER New Year's Day.

White Snowflake Party - Everyone comes dressed in white. Design a white event drink and have white snowflake decorations. This can be easily elevated to a dinner party. Give a white ornament to take home as a guest gift. Can be easily scheduled anytime around Christmas time.

Silver and Gold Party - Same as above. Easily mixed with a masquerade party.

After Christmas Regifting Party- An opportunity for guests to get rid of the things they don't want. This is a type of White Elephant Party.

New Year's Predictions Party—Bring in an Astrologer for individual readings and to see what is in store for the coming New Year.

Grilled Cheese and Soup Party- Great for a casual get-together and super easy!

Viva Las Vegas Party- Good one any time of year, but especially for the new year. Have a Best Elvis Costume contest. Play Elvis music and/or play Elvis movies.

Casino Night - Rent tables, chips, and staff. Always a fun party but needs lots of room.

Prosecco, Potato Chips, and Parmesan Party- Great as a cocktail party. Supplement with bread sticks, olives, and nuts. Super easy. Be sure to use a big chunk of good Parmesan on the food table.

Foodie Party—If your group is into fine dining, hire a local chef over and have everyone learn how it's done, or help out making dinner.

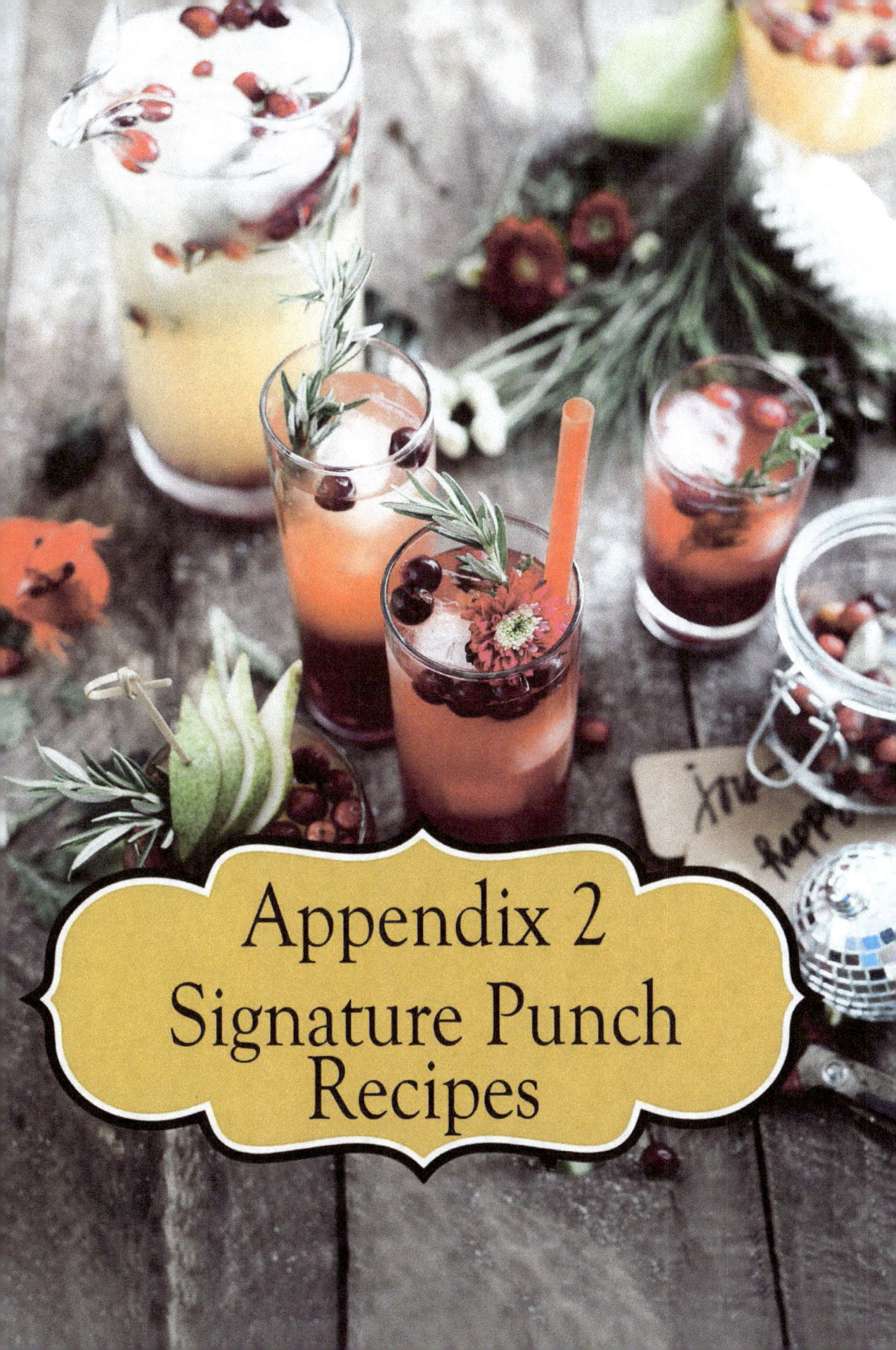

Appendix 2
Signature Punch Recipes

Signature Punch Recipes

Pineapple Mint Punch

Serves 20
Hands on time: 10 mins.
Total time: 35 mins.

1/2 cup sugar
3 quarts pineapple juice
1 liter gin
1 liter club soda
1 cup fresh lime juice
1 cup fresh mint leaves
Ice for serving

<u>Step 1</u>
Combine sugar and 1/2 cup water in a small saucepan and bring to a boil. Reduce heat and simmer until sugar dissolves. Should take 1 to 2 minutes. Let cool.
<u>Step 2</u>
In large bowl, combine sugar syrup, pineapple juice, gin, club soda, lime juice, and mint. Serve over ice.

Bourbon Ginger Snap

Serves 20
Hands on time: 10 mins.
Total time: 35 mins.

1 cup fresh lemon juice
1 cup honey
1 3-inch piece of fresh ginger, peeled and sliced
6 cups fresh orange juice
4 cups pear nectar
1 liter bourbon
2 lemons, thinly sliced
Add Ice for serving

Step 1
Combine 2 quarts water, fresh lemon juice, honey and ginger in a large saucepan and bring to a boil. Reduce heat and simmer for 5 minutes. Strain into a large bowl. Let cool.
Step 2
Add orange juice, pear nectar, bourbon, and lemons to the lemon syrup. Serve over ice.

Cranberry Cooler

Serves 20
Hands-on time: 15 mins.
Total time: 40 mins.

4 bags (12 oz. each) cranberries (fresh or frozen)
4 cups sugar
3 liters tonic
1 cup fresh lime juice
cream soda and ice

Step 1
In large saucepan combine cranberries, sugar and 2 cups water. Bring to a boil. Reduce heat and simmer for 5 minutes. Using a slotted spoon, transfer 3 cups of the cranberries to a large bowl, then strain the remaining syrup into a bowl. Let cool.
Step 2
Add the tonic water and lime juice to the cranberry syrup. Serve over ice and top off with a splash of cream soda.
Best served with vodka.

Party Punch

4 cups cran-apple juice
2 bottles red Moscato
1 bottle Prosecco
1/2 cup Vodka
2 cups frozen cranberries
1/3 cup mint leaves
1/2 cup sugar for rimming glasses
2 limes sliced in rounds

Step 1
Using a wedge of lime, wet the rim of your glasses. Dip in sugar until coated.
Step 2
Combine all ingredients in a punch bowl, stir together and serve.

Cranberry, Tangerine, and Pomegranate Punch

Serves 20
Hands-on time: 10 mins.
Total time: 40 mins.

1 bag (12 oz) fresh cranberries for swizzle sticks
1 bunch mint for swizzle sticks
2 cups pomegranate juice
3 cups tangerine juice
5 cups cranberry juice cocktail

Spear 3 cranberries alternately with 2 mint leaves on each wooden skewer. Place skewers on a baking sheet, cover with damp paper towels and refrigerate up to one hour.
In a large bowl, stir together fruit juices. Fill glasses with ice, and ladle about 1/2 cup punch into each glass. Garnish each glass with a swizzle stick.
Best served with champagne or sparkling wine.

Autumn Sangria

2-3 fresh figs and/or 1 cup dried figs (quarter or slice)
2-3 fresh plums, pitted, and/or 1 cup dried plums (prunes) cubed
1/4 cup molasses
1 750 milliliter bottle sparkling apple cider or club soda, chilled
1 orange, sliced thinly

In 3-quart glass container combine fruits and molasses; stir until mixed thoroughly. Slowly pour in red wine. Cover and chill 2-24 hours. To serve, add sparkling cider and orange. Stir. Fill glasses with ice.

Christmas and Holiday Signature Punch

Below are several recipes that can get you through numerous holiday parties. Choose the one that goes best with your theme or sounds good to you. There are no wrong choices. A punch bowl is perfect for an open house that goes on several hours. Just make sure to refresh the ice as time goes on. Frozen fruits are always festive. A candy cane to stir the drink is playful and fun.

Winter Sangria

Serves 20
Hands-on time: 20 mins.
Total time: 20 mins.

3 bottles fruity red wine such as Pinot Noir or Cabernet Sauvignon
2 liters black cherry soda
1-1/2 cups pomegranate juice
3/4 cup brandy
1/2 cup triple sec
4 pears, cored and thinly sliced
2 oranges, thinly sliced
Ice for serving

In a large bowl, combine the wine, black cherry soda, pomegranate juice, brandy, triple sec, pears, and oranges. Serve over ice.

Christmas Rum Punch

Lime slices, for ice and garnish
Apple wedges for ice and garnish
Cranberries for ice
3/4 cup Sugar
2-1/4 cups lime juice
3-3/4 cups dark rum
2-1/4 cups Grand Marnier
1-1/2 cups Amaretto
3-3/4 cups apple juice

3-1/2 cups sparkling water
Orange slices for garnish

Fill a 2-cup container with water and add lime slices, apple wedges, and cranberries. Cover and transfer to a freezer. Freeze until solid.
In a large punch bowl, combine sugar and lime juice until dissolved. Add rum, Grand Marnier, Amaretto, and apple juice. Transfer to refrigerator until ready to serve.
Add ice and top with sparkling water. Garnish with lime slices, orange slices, apple wedges, and cinnamon.

Santa's Favorite Christmas Punch

2 cups chilled unsweetened pomegranate juice
1 cup chilled cranberry juice
1 cup Vodka
1 cup Cointreau (orange flavor liqueur)
1 cup chilled club soda
1/2 cup fresh lemon juice (2 or 3)
1/2 cup simple syrup for mixed drinks
Cranberries frozen in ice cubes

Chill pomegranate juice, cranberry juice, club soda before starting. Combine pomegranate and cranberry juice, vodka, Cointreau, club soda, lemon juice, and simple syrup in a punch bowl. Fill glasses with cranberries frozen in ice cubes and serve.

Christmas Sangria

2 cups cranberry juice
1 cup fresh squeezed clementine or orange juice
2 bottles dry red wine
1/2 cup sugar
Orange slices, clementines, fresh or frozen cranberries, fresh raspberries or halved strawberries, lemon slices, and other cut up fruit
Ice cubes

In a 3-quart pitcher or punch bowl stir together cranberry juice and clementine juice. Add wine and sugar, stirring until sugar dissolves. Cover; chill for at least 3 hours or up to 24 hours to blend flavors. Stir in fruit before serving. Serve over ice.

Open House Punch

This is a very easy recipe for Southern Comfort fans!

1 cup Southern Comfort
1 cup cranberry juice
3 oz. lemon juice
24 oz. Squirt or Wink

Serves 8 to 10 4 oz. servings.

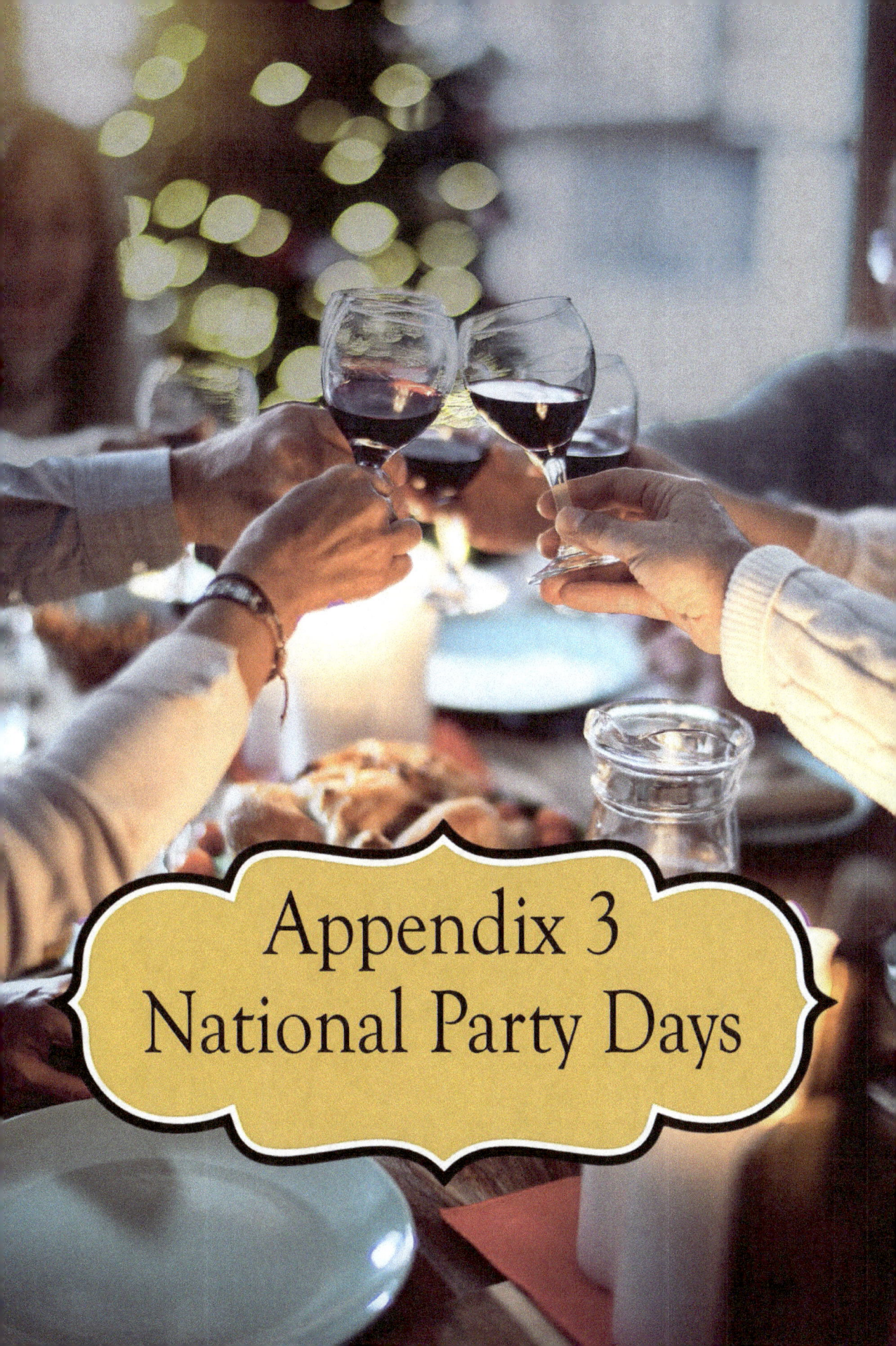

Appendix 3
National Party Days

List of National Party Days

There are so many reasons and opportunities for parties year-round. An Easter Brunch, a Fourth of July barbeque, St. Patrick's Day, Kentucky Derby.

In January, plan out your entire year's entertaining schedule. Three to four events a year is normal.

Put tentative dates on your calendar and start enjoying your entertaining skills! Be creative! Find any reason to have a party—National Ice Cream Day? Have an ice cream party with alcohol flavors. There are so many reasons to celebrate!

The website www.nationaltoday.com lists 116 days in January alone! If you want to entertain, finding a "hook" is easy. Feel free to check out their website. It's a great place to find a reason to have a party.

Note: Some holidays are on a different date every year. For instance, Thanksgiving and Chinese New Year are figured differently each year. Those dates are starred (**).

I have also made some comments on how you can develop the ideas.

January

1 **National Bloody Mary Day**
National Hangover Day
New Year's Day
A trifecta to celebrate! These naturally go together for a cozy afternoon of watching football with friends and family. Keep it easy—chips and dips, maybe a delicious pot of chili to help keep warm in colder climes.

3   **National Mind-Body Wellness Day**
     This one could be an interesting ladies' day. Maybe have a nutritionist come in and speak to your guests. Or bring in a manicurist, perhaps, someone to do massages or facials, anything to support pampering. Champagne and salads would be appropriate food. Everyone should bring their robes and slippers!

4   **National Spaghetti Day**
     Supply the noodles and let guests bring their favorite sauce, hopefully already hot to avoid stove congestion. You supply the crunchy bread, breadsticks and salad. It's nice to have two or three kinds of noodles. Perhaps use a spaghetti noodle, penne, and maybe a cheese ravioli. Don't forget the parmesan cheese Decorate with the Italian flag, play Italian music. Some chianti, or prosecco for drinks. Maybe some cannoli for dessert.

8   **National Elvis Birthday Day**
     There's lots of ways to go including asking guests to come in their favorite Elvis outfit! Play Elvis movies and play music for sure. A dance floor would be nice. Could incorporate a 50's look. Poodle skirts and black and white oxfords?

9   **National Cheese Lover's Day**
     Cheese is the workhorse and hero of parties! Have you ever gone to a party that did not have some kind of cheese? Its versatility is what makes it special. Cheese can be in appetizers, in a salad, the main course, or dessert. How about a party celebrating cheese where everyone brings their favorite cheese recipe? Now, if this date corresponds with a Green Bay Packers game, you have a perfect match for cheese head fans.

27   **National Chocolate Cake Day**
     Who doesn't love chocolate? This is a versatile day for either a Ladies' Day or a couples' dessert party. Everyone can bring their favorite chocolate cake! You supply some fruit to counter the richness, nice dessert plates, maybe whipped cream or ice cream. Champagne or Champagne punch would be nice. Maybe have some coffee available. This would also work if you went out earlier for dinner or for a concert and have everyone come back to your house. You supply a few different choices of cake, plug in the coffee, and pop the

champagne. Setting up napkins and glasses before you leave for the earlier event, makes this a very easy party with minimal preparation.

February

** **Chinese New Year**
Do a little research and match your guests with the appropriate Chinese astrological sign which is based on month and year of your birth. You can order Chinese food from your local favorite restaurant or have a Chinese menu you prepare. This holiday has many traditions and I urge you to learn them and share them with your guests.

** **Superbowl**
My son was born on Super Bowl Sunday, and we always had a big party with friends and family. It was our tradition to have a big pot of meaty chili available through the afternoon. There was a big bowl of grated cheese and chopped onions to put on top. Of course, chips, dips, and cut veggies. Cheese quesadillas were an easy addition. It is a long day, and menu planning depends on making food last over many hours. It's fun to have some wagering, and a lively crowd. We even had a contest for best commercials! Very warm memories.

14 **Valentine's Day**
If you have a tight group of couples, this can be a nice night with a formal dinner. With so many other reasons to have a party, this might just be one to avoid and spend with your significant other. It is however, not a bad night to have a party for just singles. Valentine's Day is not a favorite of Singles, so a party might just be the ticket.

18 **National Drink Wine Day**
You could have a wine tasting? Set out some grapes, fruit, crackers, breadsticks, and different cheeses. Have lots of glasses. Perhaps, plan for some designated drivers?

22 **National Margarita Day**
Bring out the Mexican hats, chips, and guacamole, maybe some tacos, and fire up the blender. Just like National Drink Wine Day, designated drivers are recommended!

March

**   **Mardi Gras**

The pageantry and tradition in Mardi Gras are always fun. Fat Tuesday is usually a big party night. Do some research about all the customs like the King Cake and Mardi Gras costumes. Perhaps you can have fun masks, beads, even New Orleans Jazz music. Be creative!

17   **St. Patrick's Day**

You don't have to be Irish to celebrate St. Patrick's Day! Encourage your guests to wear green and dress to celebrate the holiday. Lots of green beer, corned beef and cabbage brings it all together. You might take turns reading some Irish limericks. Play some Irish music to enhance the mood.

20   **Spring Equinox**

Have a gardening party and your guests can go home with some freshly planted flowers. This is a good lunch party.

26   **National Wear a Hat Day**

Have prizes for the most outlandish. A photo booth would be fun, too. Perfectly suited for a brunch or afternoon party.

April

1   **April Fool's Day**

This can be fun but takes some planning. Great with the right crowd.

6   **National Walking Day**

This is a party planned with the weather in mind. A beautiful sunset walk in the Spring is a particular treat. You can plan a menu that you can put on hold, and everyone can go on a nice walk before the party begins.

7   **National Beer Day**
      National Burrito Day

This is an easy pairing! Burritos can be assembled ahead of time and are a good menu choice. Add salad, chips, and guacamole. How about a craft beer tasting?

12	**National Grilled Cheese Sandwich Day**

I've included this as this was one of my Mother's favorite parties. It's an easy one because you can make the sandwiches ahead of time and keep them warm in the oven, making them even more gooey. Cut into fourths for easy finger food. Try using some different cheeses for an assortment. Monterey Jack, Havarti, Cheddar, and Swiss all work. Mom used to love grilled cheddar and slices of apple. Have some baskets of potato chips, and some bread and butter pickles. You could even make some tomato soup for real comfort food.

** Easter

This is one of my favorite holidays to have a brunch. Brunches are often overlooked in party planning, and a brunch has so many possibilities. You do need to get up earlier in the morning, but much of the preparation can be done the day before. And clean-up is usually completed before dark; maybe leaving time for a peaceful and well-deserved afternoon nap. Easter is so much fun and is a very uplifting holiday and is perfect suited for a well-planned brunch. Decorations are fun and whimsical; the promise of Spring brings everyone closer. Add in some Mimosas and Bloody Mary's and it makes for a very lazy, beautiful afternoon.

May

1 May Day

There are many traditions regarding May Day. Do some research and share it with your guests. Spring hats would be fun.

5 Cinco de Mayo

While this is more of an American holiday than a Mexican party, it does play well in party planning with lots of menu items and everyone loves Margaritas! How about a tequila tasting?

7 National Beer Pong Day

** Kentucky Derby

It doesn't take much imagination in putting these two together! I've had several students plan Kentucky Derby Parties. It can be a long day, even though the actual race is less than 5 minutes long. Lots of chances for fun wagering, fun hats, and mint juleps. Do some research on other customs of this famous race.

13 **National Apple Pie Day**
Have your guests bring their favorite recipes to share with the other guests. Have a blind apple pie tasting test with awards.

14 **National Dance Like a Chicken Day**
I just had to include this one. You can use your imagination on how to put this together. You could have a dance contest. You can serve lots of chicken dishes. Deviled Eggs. I think there should probably be alcohol involved. Best for a lively group comfortable with each other.

20 **National Nascar Day**
National Pizza Party Day
If you have a group that enjoy NASCAR races, your menu is already taken care of with National Pizza party day!

24 **National Scavenger Hunt Day**
Scavenger hunts in golf carts are a hoot! Make boxed lunches with easy finger foods for the Hunt. Have dessert at your house after your adventure with awards.

June

11 **National King Kamehameha Day**
Perfect day for a luau! Especially nice if you have a pool. Play Hawaiian music, serve mai tais, and don't forget the little umbrellas!

17 **National Flip Flop Day**
National Root Beer Day
These 2 could work well together. How about root beer floats? And I'm sure there is some alcoholic drink that would incorporate root beer.

18 **International Picnic Day**
There are some beautiful areas in most communities for a picnic. Whether for lunch or dinner, it's a nice, casual way to enjoy friends. Try to time dessert for evening time and toast the setting sun!

** **Father's Day**

19 **National Martini Day**
Sometimes it's great to put two holidays together.

20	**National Ice Cream Soda Day**
	National Milkshake Day

These two can easily work together. How about a 50's soda fountain party complete with poodle skirts and spin some rock and roll and have some dancing?

21	**Summer Solstice**

Celebrate the beginning of Summer!

July

4	**Independence Day**

The Fourth of July has always been one of my favorite holidays. Usually the weather is glorious, the flowers are in bloom, and everyone becomes enveloped in traditions and patriotism. The reward of fireworks at the end of the day makes for great memories. Great day to fire up the barbecue!

6	**International Kissing Day**
	National Fried Chicken Day

Good excuse for a potluck? Everyone brings their favorite fried chicken dish. How to integrate International Kissing Day is totally up to you!

7	**National Strawberry Sundae Day**
	World Chocolate Day
8	**National Chocolate with Almonds Day**
9	**National Sugar Cookie Day**

These 3 days can be celebrated together for a true sugar high!

10	**National Pina Colada Day**

This could be integrated with a luau theme. Or a Caribbean theme complete with steel drums.

11	**Cheer Up the Lonely Day**
	National Mojito Day

After quarantine and the pandemic, there are probably many who have felt the loneliness of isolation. What better way to pick up spirits with National Mojito Day? Bring in some Cuban food?

14	**Bastille Day**
	National Mac and Cheese Day
	National Nude Day

I had a French friend and Bastille Day Parties were always a treat!

19   **National Daiquiri Day**
     This could be a fun tasting party sampling different kinds of daiquiris.
24   **National Day of the Cowboy**
     National Tequila Day
     Everyone comes dressed in Western Wear and have a tequila tasting? There are so many kinds of tequila and doing some research ahead of time and sharing with your guests the intricacies of tequila making would be fun.

27   **National Scotch Day**
     Scotch making is art. Invest in a few bottles of unusual scotch, get some cigars, and play cards or board games.
29   **National Chicken Wing Day**
     National Chili Dog Day
     National Lasagna Day
     I guess the menu is easy on this one!

August

1   **National Friendship Day**
     National Girlfriend Day
     What a great day to get together with old friends and new friends!
3   **National Watermelon Day**
     National White Wine Day
     Tom Brady's Birthday
     If Tom Brady is very popular in your area., why not have a birthday cake for him? You can also celebrate the other 2 days at the same time. National Watermelon Day and National White Wine Day sounds refreshing! Integrate the watermelon into your menu with a watermelon salsa or a watermelon signature drink to mix with the white wine. Have several choices of white wine and have a taste test.
6   **International Beer Day**
     National Beer Float Day
     If you have friends who enjoy their beer, this is a party for them!
18   **National Couples Day**
     National Fajita Day

You might be in a group of friends who are couples and enjoy doing things together! Celebrate your friendship! Fajitas are not a difficult menu item!

19   **National Potato Day**

One of my students had a potato party and was so creative. Potato soup, potato pancakes, french fries, and a chubby Mr. Potato head decoration.

28   **National Bow Tie Day**
       National Red Wine Day

Invite EVERYONE to wear a bow tie! Have a variety of red wines for tasting.

September

**   **Labor Day**

A great day signaling the end of Summer. Snowbirds will be returning soon.

5   **International Day of Charity**

A great opportunity to give back and have a party at the same time. Have your guests bring canned goods for the food bank, school supplies for the local schools, items for the homeless shelter.

7   **National Wiener Schnitzel Day**

A party to celebrate your German heritage or that of your neighbors. Add in some German music, beer, sauerkraut, and some lederhosen and you have a party. Why wait until Oktoberfest??

21   **National Miniature Golf Day**

There may be miniature golf courses in your area. Why not meet everyone there and come back to your house for dessert or happy hour?

25   **National Lobster Day**

If your pocketbook can handle it, a lobster feast is always fun. Get some butcher paper for your outside dining table, steam the lobster, warm some butter, cut up a lemon, a good loaf of bread and you have a party. You could also do a New England boil and include other shellfish, potatoes, and corn.

28   **National Neighbor Day**

This is definitely worth celebrating and truly contributes to building a sense of community. It's time again to make lifelong friends with your neighbors.

October

1   **International Music Day**

If you are into music, seek out symbiotic friends in your area. Celebrate and share the music you love and that makes your soul sing!

4   **National Golf Lovers Day**
National Taco Day
National Vodka Day

Another trifecta! This is an easy one!

10   **National Cake Decorating Day**

A fun way to spend the afternoon! Have everyone bring their own cooled cakes and have all the frosting, piping bags, and cake decorations ready to go. If you can locate a local baker for a demonstration, even better!

14   **National I Love Lucy Day**

This could be a really fun party! Have some I love Lucy shows running, have some trivia games ready. Serve food from the 50's and encourage costumes.

31   **Halloween**

In the pre-pandemic years, Halloween was a perfect time for parties. One year I wore four different costumes! If you are planning on a Halloween party, make sure your invitations go out early as it is a very popular time of the year. It's also a natural for theme and decorations. Always make sure to have a Photo Booth so everyone has a souvenir!

November

11   **Veterans Day**

This is a very special day and there are veterans in every community. This is a special day to honor them.

SECRETS OF STRESS-FREE ENTERTAINING

** **Thanksgiving**
You may have family visiting or you may plan on visiting them. If you are staying home, I would encourage you to increase your guest list to those that may not have a place to go or may not have someone. Holidays can be a very hard time of the year and including them will exemplify what Thanksgiving is all about. Don't forget to donate to the food bank so that those less fortunate can celebrate Thanksgiving as well. Remember your local food bank throughout the year.

** **National Black Friday Day**

26 **National Cake Day**
Spending money and Christmas shopping online with your friends while eating cake? Why not?? Sounds like fun! Let the games begin!

December

December is a very busy month for most people. Plan early to reserve the date of your event. Consider a "save the date" card if you are still in the development stage.

1 **National Christmas Lights Day**
There is nothing that signals the Holidays more than lighting up our houses! Why not make it an annual event with your immediate neighbors to help each other get it all set up? Maybe the group could help out any of those that can't physically put up the decorations in your neighborhood. It's a great bonding event for your community. After the lights are all up, light them all up at the same time and have a driveway party to celebrate!

9 **National Christmas Card Day**
National Pastry Day
The art of handwriting Christmas cards is becoming a lost tradition. How about spending an afternoon writing out some Christmas cards, while enjoying an assortment of pastries? You could also piggyback this with a Christmas wrapping party where everyone can help each other get it all done? Or writing Christmas wishes to service members stationed overseas?

18 **National Bake Cookies Day**
Have a group event or do a cookie swap.

20   **National Go Caroling Day**
     National Sangria Day
     What a great community activity! The sharing of voices is always fun. And pairing it with National Sangria Day is brilliant!

24   **Christmas Eve**
     If you are staying home for the holidays, Christmas Eve is the perfect time to drop off a small gift to your neighbors; especially those that might be alone. Time is the most valuable gift you can give another.

28   **Cardplaying Day**
     Chocolate Candy Day
     A fun day to kick back and recover from the holidays.

31   **New Year's Eve**
     National Champagne Day
     New Year's Eve is a perfect night for an intimate dinner party. Dress up, share a nice meal with champagne and toast the new year. However, plan on a late clean-up.

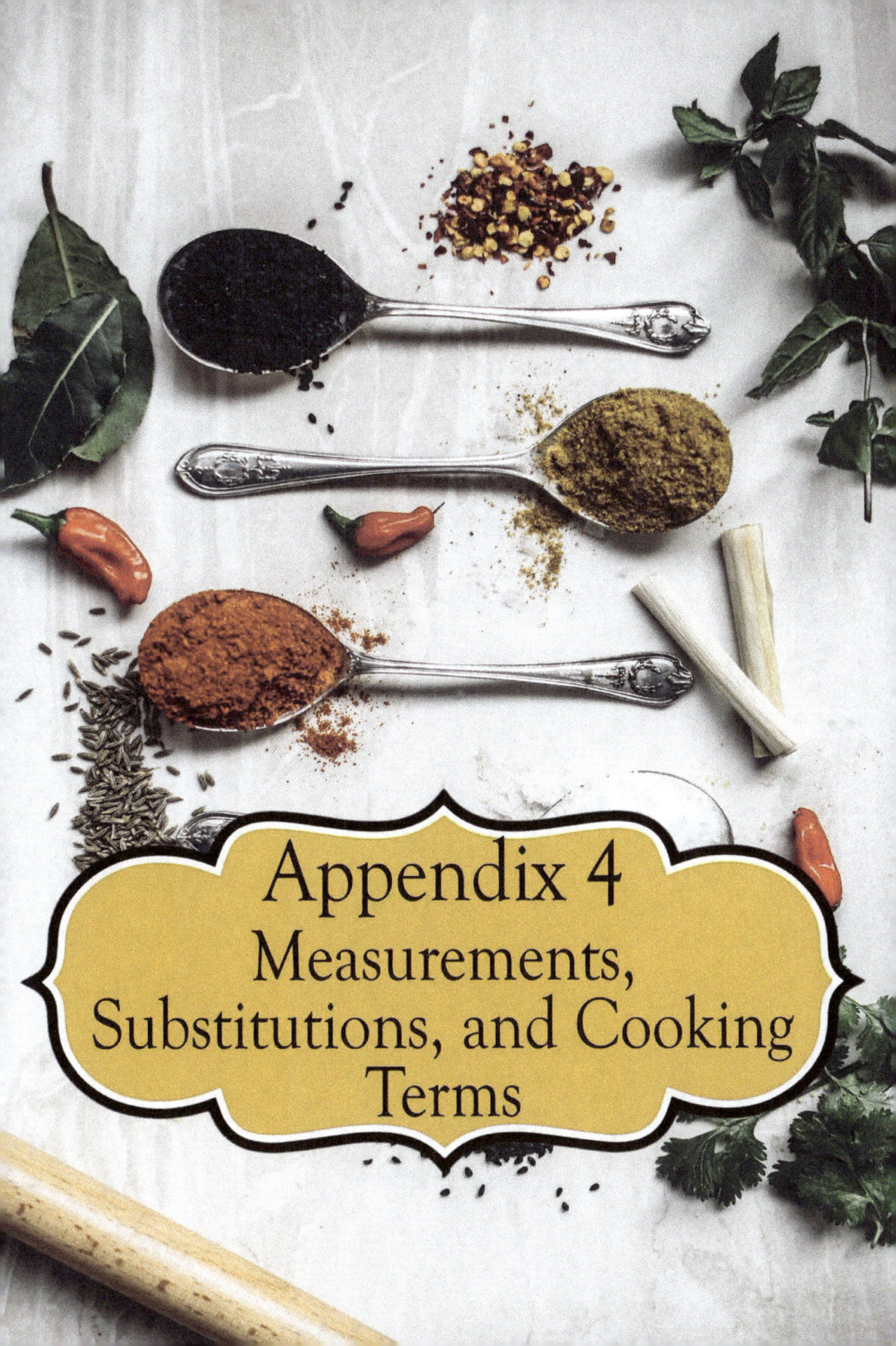

Appendix 4
Measurements, Substitutions, and Cooking Terms

Measurements, Equivalents, Substitutions, and Cooking Terms

I'm including this list because it's usually at the last minute that you realize that you have forgotten an ingredient or are just a little short on something. Keep these handy!

Food Equivalents

	Recipe	Equivalent
Grains		
Macaroni	1 cup (3 1/2 oz). uncooked	2 1/2 cups cooked
Noodle, Med.	3 cups (4 oz.) uncooked	4 cups cooked
Popcorn	1/3 to 1/2 cup unpeopled	8 cups popped
Rice, Long Grain	1 cup uncooked	3 cups cooked
Rice, Quick Cooking	1 cup uncooked	2 cups cooked
Spaghetti	8 oz. uncooked	4 cups cooked
Crumbs		
Bread	1 slice	3/4 cup. soft /1/4 cup fine
Graham Crackers	7 squares	1/2 cup finely crushed
Round crackers	12 crackers	1/2 cup finely crushed
Saltine Crackers	14 crackers	1/2 cup finely crushed
Fruit		
Banana	1 medium	1/3 cup mashed
Lemon/Lime	1 medium	3 tbs. juice 2 tsp grated peel
Orange	1 medium	1/4-1/3 cup juice, 4 tsp. grated peel
Vegetables		
Cabbage	1 head	5 cups shredded
Carrots	1 pound	3 cups shredded
Celery	1 rib	1/2 cup. chopped
Corn	1 ear fresh	2/3 cup kernels
Green Pepper	1 large	1 cup chopped
Mushrooms	1/2 pound	3 cups sliced
Onions	1 medium	1/2 cup. chopped
Potatoes	3 medium	2 cups cubed
Nuts		
Almonds	1 pound	3 cups chopped
Ground Nuts	3-3/4 oz.	1 cup
Pecan Halves	1 pound	4-1/2 c. chopped
Walnuts	1 pound	3-3/4 chopped

Equivalent Measures

3 teaspoons	1 tablespoon
4 tablespoons	1/4 cup
5-1/3 tablespoons	1/3 cup
8 tablespoons	1/2 cup
16 tablespoons	1 cup
2 cups	1 pint
4 cups	1 quart
4 quarts	1 gallon

Easy Substitutions

When you need		Use
Baking Powder	1 teaspoon	1/2 tsp. cream of tartar plus 1/4 tsp. baking soda
Buttermilk	1 cup	1 tbsp. lemon juice or vinegar plus milk to measure 1 cup. Let stand 5 minutes before using.
Cornstarch	1 tablespoon	2 tbsp. all-purpose flour
Honey	1 cup	1-1/4 cups sugar plus 1/4 cup water
Half and half cream	1 cup	1 tbsp. melted butter plus milk to measure one cup
Onion	1 small chopped	1 tsp. onion powder or 1 tbsp diced dried onion
Tomato Juice	1 cup	1/2 cup tomato sauce plus 1/2 cup water
Tomato Sauce	2 cups	3/4 cup tomato paste plus 1 cup water
Unsweetened chocolate	1 square (1 oz.)	3 tbs. baking cocoa plus 1 tbsp. shortening or oil
Whole Milk	1 cup	1/2 cup evaporated milk plus 1/2 cup water

Cooking Terms

I know some of these are basic, but I want to make this book as inclusive as possible for all levels of kitchen expertise.

Baste
To moisten food with melted butter, pan drippings, marinades, or other liquid to add more flavor and juiciness.

Beat
A rapid movement to combine ingredients using a fork, spoon, wire whisk or electric mixer.

Blend
To combine ingredients until just mixed.

Boil
To heat liquids until bubbles form that cannot be stirred down. In the case of water, the temperature will reach 212 degrees.

Bone
To remove all meat from the bone before cooking.

Cream
To beat ingredients together to a smooth consistency, usually in the case of butter and sugar for baking.

Dash
A small amount of seasoning, less than 1/8 teaspoon. If using a shaker, a dash would comprise a quick flip of the container.

Dredge
To coat foods with flour or other dry ingredients. Most often done with pot roasts and stew meat before browning.

Fold
To incorporate several ingredients by careful and gentle turning with a spatula. Used generally with beaten egg whites or whipped cream when mixing into the rest of the ingredients to keep the batter light.

Julienne
To cut foods into long thin strips much like matchsticks. Used most often for salads and stir fry dishes.

Mince
To cut into very fine pieces. Used often for garlic or fresh herbs.

Parboil
To cook partially, usually used in the case of chicken, sausages, and vegetables.

Partially Set
Describes the consistency of gelatin after it has been chilled for a small amount of time. Mixture should resemble the consistency of egg whites.

Puree
To process foods to a smooth mixture. Can be prepared in an electric blender, food processor, food mill or sieve.

Sauté
To fry quickly in a small amount of fat, stirring almost constantly. Most often done with onions, mushrooms, and other chopped vegetables.
Score
To cut slits partway through the outer surface of foods. Often used with ham or flank steak.
Stir-Fry
To cook meats and/or vegetables with a constant stirring motion in a small amount of oil in a wok or skillet over high heat.

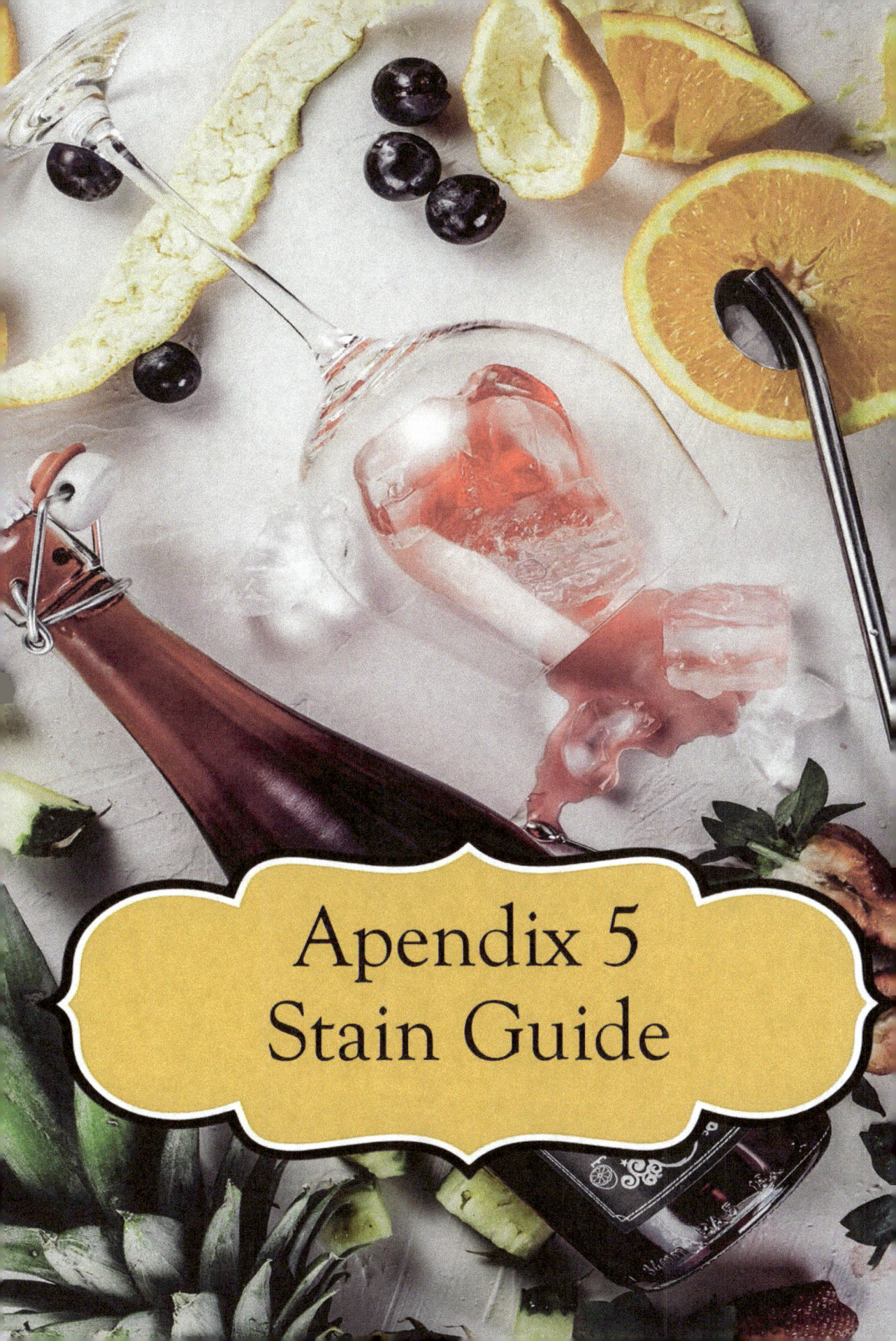

Apendix 5
Stain Guide

Stain Guide

There are always accidents. Below is a stain guide you can use when there is an "oops" moment in your entertaining adventures.

Food Grease
Let it sit in dish soap for 10 minutes before laundering with cold water. Repeat if necessary. Confirm stain is gone before putting it in dryer.

Pumpkin and Sweet Potato
Scrape off any excess and run the fabric inside out under cold water. Pretreat with a laundry stain remover, then wash fabric on hot.

Cranberry Sauce
Rinse the stain with cool water. Add 1 tbs. white vinegar and 1/2 tsp. liquid laundry detergent to one-quart cold water. Blot the mixture on the stain with a clean cloth until it disappears.

Candle Wax
Scrape what you can with a dull knife. Use a hairdryer to melt remaining wax. This will leave an oily residue that can be dabbed away with a cotton ball soaked in rubbing alcohol. Launder item as usual.

Chocolate
Remove any crumbs or hardened chocolate with a dry, clean toothbrush. Add 1 tbs. dish soap to 2 cups warm water and apply the mixture using a microfiber cloth, dabbing the stain. Do not rub. Repeat a few times before soaking the solution with a clean towel.

Gravy
Add 1/4 tsp. dishwashing liquid and 3 cups ammonia to 1/2 cup warm water. Using a clean cloth, press the solution into the stain but do not rub. If the spill is on silk or wool, use club soda instead of ammonia.

Lipstick
Pretreat with liquid laundry detergent, working it in with a toothbrush. Should sit for at least 15 minutes then wash fabric on hot. If necessary, repeat before putting in dryer

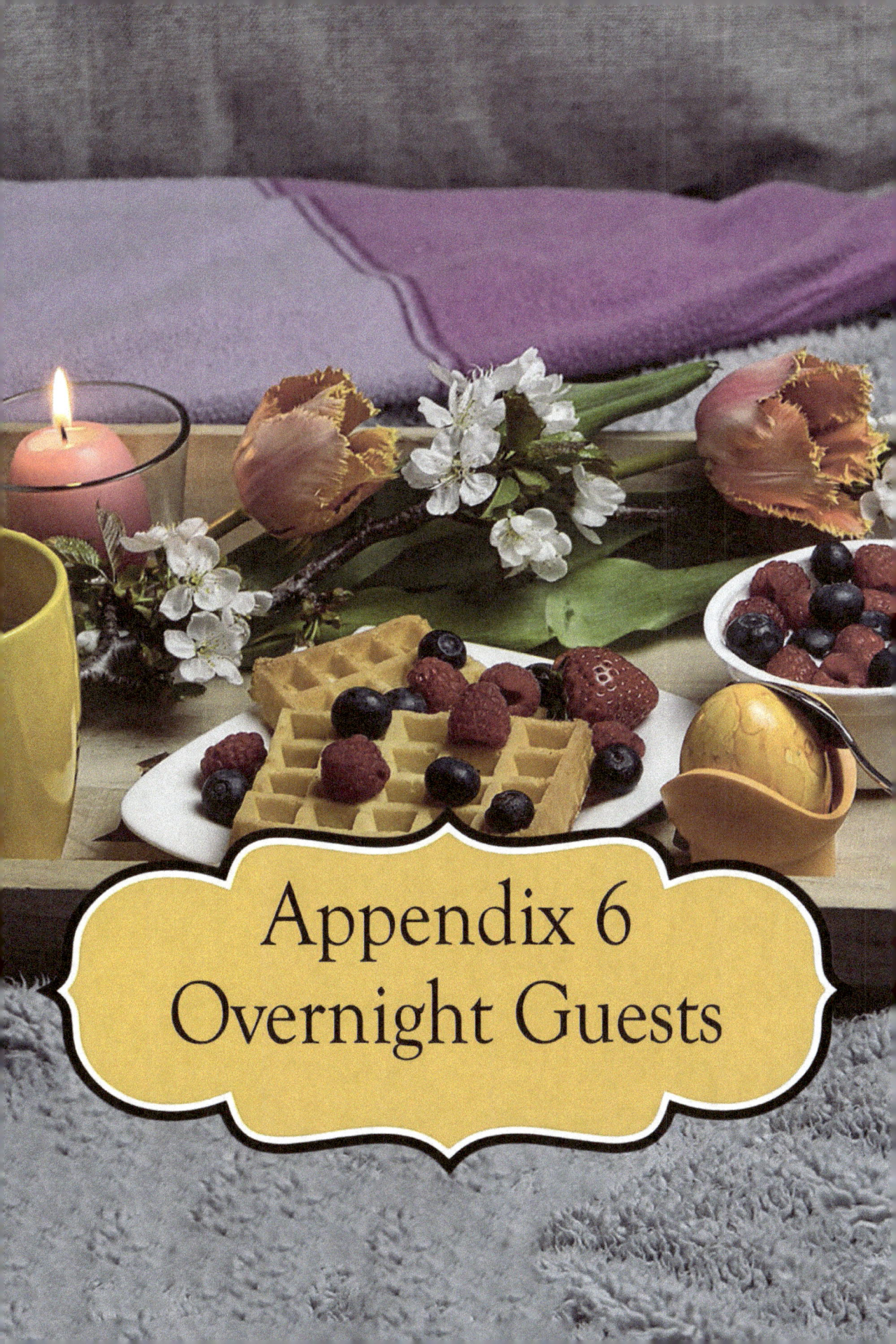

Appendix 6
Overnight Guests

Overnight Guests

Overnight guests present some unique hosting challenges. What's most important is knowing their expectations and communicating yours. Ask your guests before their arrival what they would like to do. Are they looking forward to some relaxation, or are they anticipating around-the-clock activities?

Some tips

1. Know the number of meals you will be eating at home. Plan the meals that you will be serving ahead of time. Make a list for each meal including each ingredient you will need to buy.

2. Have lots of food available in the refrigerator for snacking. I like to make things up before guests arrive that are easy and which everyone likes. Sometimes you may be on a different time zone; it can take a few days before people are all hungry at the same time.

Some foods I like to have on hand include a fruit salad, which can work for breakfast or anytime during the day. Also, your best potato salad and pasta salad works well. Have a variety of lunchmeat and sliced cheeses for quick sandwiches. Include a couple of different kinds of breads: white, rye, and whole wheat are favorites.

3. Find out what your guests like to drink and stock up.

4. Make sure the bed linens are clean and prepared before any overnight guests arrive.

5. Make sure your guests have access to clean towels, without rummaging through your cluttered linen closet. You might reserve some newer towels just for guests.
6. Put out some local reading material in their room including magazines.

7. Have a few bottles of water, maybe some wrapped candies, or some cookies in a nice basket.

8. Put out sample bottles of shampoo, conditioner, a disposable razor, mouthwash, a new toothbrush, and toothpaste. I also like to keep a bottle of Tylenol and Pepto Bismol in the guest medicine chest.

9. Avoid politics and religion in conversations.

10. Plan things for your guests and you to do together; it's always best discussed before they arrive. It lets people know what to pack and adds to their trip anticipation.

11. Make any necessary reservations and ticket purchases before they arrive

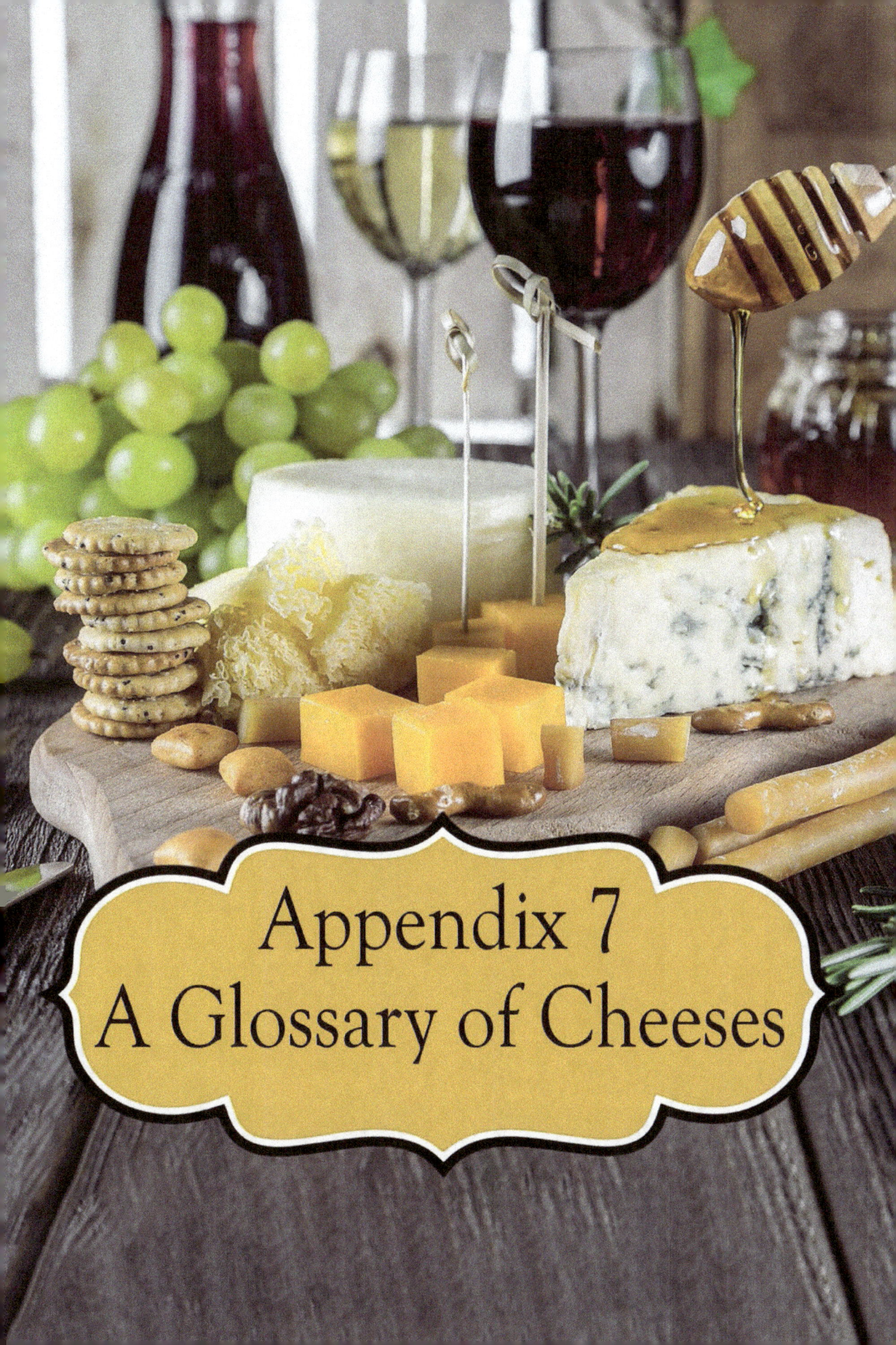

Appendix 7
A Glossary of Cheeses

A Glossary of Cheeses

Asiago

Made from cow's milk, this exotic cheese is prepared only in the Asiago region of Italy. As it matures, the cheese changes in texture and taste; while fresh Asiago is softer, the aged variants are more susceptible to falling apart. The rind may also vary in color, some being brownish gray, while others take on a straw-colored hue. Asiago cheese has about 48 percent fat and is usually grated onto salads and sandwiches.

Brie

Brie is the best-known French cheese and is nicknamed "The Queen of Cheeses." This soft cheese is named after the French region of Brie, where it was originally created. Several years ago, Brie was one of the tributes which had to be paid to the French kings.

While Brie is produced from whole or semi-skimmed cow's milk, rennet is added into raw milk and heated to a temperature of 37 degrees C. to obtain the curd. This cheese is then cast into molds of several layers and kept for 18 hours. From there, the cheese is salted and aged for a minimum of four weeks.

Brie cheese is slightly pale in color with a grayish tinge under its rind. Brie goes well with champagne, nuts, and fruit, or can be used as a dessert. The white, soft rind is a mold growth, a form of penicillin, to be exact. In some circles, the rind alone is considered a delicacy. Sweet and pillowy soft, it complements the cheese well. It is this rind that gives the cheese its gooey goodness. Over time, the live rind breaks down the fats and proteins in the cheese, causing an increasingly creamy-to-runny texture.

Camembert

Camembert is a rare type of cheese first manufactured in Normandy, France. Not many are adept in the techniques required to produce this cheese, hence, there are only a handful of manufacturers of its kind. The most exquisite of all Camembert cheeses is the Camembert Le Chatelain. This cheese is like the wine that usually accompanies: the older, the better. As it ages, its texture becomes creamier and tastes more buttery.

Cheddar

Cheddar Cheese is a relatively hard, off-white cheese (or orange, if colorings such as annatto are added.) It is sometimes a sharp-tasting, natural cheese. Cheddar originated in the English village of Cheddar in Somerset; cheeses of this style are now produced around the world. Outside of Europe, the style and quality of cheeses labeled as Cheddar may vary greatly, with some processed cheeses being packaged as "Cheddar" while bearing little resemblance. Furthermore, certain cheeses that are more similar in taste and appearance to Red Leicester are sometimes popularly marketed as "red Cheddar."

Chevre

This is a French classic example of goat's cheese, which hits the right note with people who do not care much for cow's milk. It is quite healthy owing to its high potassium and vitamin qualities and low-fat content. The earthy taste makes it a highly popular cheese not just in France, but in many other countries. Ideally, Chèvre should be soft and mushy enclosed in a harder exterior. This cheese makes for an excellent companion for wine and other spirits.

Cotija

Several decades ago, Mexico introduced the world to the famous Cotija cheese. This salty cheese tastes as good as Parmesan, and is crumbly in texture, thus making it easier to use as a garnish. It takes about three to 12 months to prepare this cheese. Freshly prepared Cotija has a mushy texture but achieves a harder textural quality as it matures.

Emmenthal

This is a Swiss delicacy, which is tough to prepare, but quite easy to recognize, because of the number of holes, formed after its fermentation. The Emmenthal, which is hard in texture, tastes rich and fruity and perfectly complements a glass of wine. (Also see Swiss cheese.)

Feta

A white, salty, sharp-tasting cheese made from sheep's or goat's milk, with a crumbly, creamy to dry consistency. It's a favorite of Greece and Greek dishes. It is accepted as unadulterated only if it has been produced in Thessaly, Macedonia, Lesvos, Thrace, the Peloponnese, and Central Mainland Greece. If it is made somewhere else, it is called "white cheese." This cheese, which matures after a period of two months, is made from goat's milk and is usually squishy in texture, although certain kinds may be a bit more crumbly.

Fontina

Firm, creamy, delicate Italian cheese with a slightly nutty taste; made from cow's milk. Look for Fontina from the Aosta Valley of northwestern Italy. The Fontina d'Aosta dates to the 12th century when it was first produced in Italy; its rind gains an orange-brown tint as it matures over a period of time. Depending on the age of the cheese, the Fontina may range in texture and taste. It is savored as a suitable snack with red wine, apart from being used in cakes and desserts.

Goat Cheese

Most cheeses made from goat's milk are fresh and creamy, with a distinctive sharp tang. They are sometimes coated with pepper, ash, or herbs, which mellows them. It is also known by the French as Chèvre.

Gorgonzola

A creamy, blue-veined Italian cheese. This Italian masterpiece is an absolute visual delight with blue veins running across the entire surface of the cheese. A popular cheese, it is soft and crumbly with a nutty flavor. It can take up to four months to mature, and depending on its age, the varieties can be Gorgonzola Piccante or Gorgonzola Dolce. Other creamy blue cheeses may be substituted.

Gouda

Gouda is a mild, yellow cheese, hard to semi-hard, originating from the Netherlands and made from cow's milk. It is one the most popular cheeses worldwide. The name is used today as a general term for numerous similar cheeses produced in the traditional Dutch manner.

Gruyere

This is a type of Swiss cheese with a firm, smooth texture, small holes, and relatively strong flavor.

Manchego

This Spanish cheese is a product of sheep's milk and takes a period of three to 12 months to age. Depending on the time period it is fermented, the variants could be the Semi-Curado, Curado, or Viejo. The youngest Manchego is fruity in flavor, while the oldest tastes sweet. This winner of the 2014 World Cheese Awards, stand out from the crowd, because of its rich taste and the basketweave design on its surface.
Mexican Manchego cheese is made from cow or sheep's milk.

Mascarpone

Mascarpone cheese looks more like thick cream, which is the base ingredient for its preparation. An Italian creation, it is acidic because of the lime added to it and is high in fat owing to its use of full-fat cream.

The Mascarpone is widely used in cheesecakes and scones, or with fresh fruits. However, its robust flavors do not last for a long time. It needs to be consumed within days of preparation, or else it may go stale.

Monterey Jack

A semisoft white melting cheese with a mild flavor and buttery texture. Pepper Jack is a spicy cousin.

Mozzarella

Rindless white, mild-tasting Italian cheese traditionally made from water buffalo's milk and sold fresh. Commercially produced and packaged cow's milk mozzarella is more common, but less flavorful. Look for fresh mozzarella packed in water.

Parmesan

Hard, thick crusted aged Italian cow's milk cheese with a sharp, salty, full flavor. The finest Italian variety is designated Parmigiano-Reggiano. Buy in block form, to grate fresh as needed.

Pecorino Toscano

The Pecorino Toscano (famous by the name" Toscanello") is another Italian gastronomical delight. Produced by local farmers of Tuscany, this cheese is sweet and nutty and is reminiscent of a decadent dessert. Ideally, the Toscanello should be enjoyed with a sweet fruit like the apple.

Provolone

Italians have given us some of the most delicious treats on earth: pizza, pasta, and of course, cheese. Provolone is one of those cheeses that one must absolutely taste. The lighter Provolone Dolce takes about three months to age. Provolone Piccante, as the name suggests, is more piquant in flavor and takes more than four months to mature. This cheese goes best with bread, meat, and wine.

Ricotta

Fresh Italian cheese made by heating the whey left over from making other cheeses. Traditionally based on sheep's milk, however, today's cow's milk ricotta is more common in most food stores.

Robiola Piemonte

This is one of the most luxurious cheeses ever made by the Italians. A mixture of sheep, cow, and goat's milk is used to manufacture this delectable cheese. It is so vibrant in flavor that it's most commonly used as a table cheese that can be relished with a dash of salt and pepper.

Roquefort

This French cheese, which takes approximately five months to age, became famous because it struck the right chord with Emperor Charlemagne. The reason it is so popular in France and elsewhere is because of its richness and its multilayered flavors.

Swiss

Swiss Cheese is a generic name in North America for several related varieties of cheese; a yellow, medium-hard cheese that originated in the area around Emmental, in Switzerland. Some types of Swiss Cheese have a distinctive appearance, as the blocks of cheese are riddled with holes, known as "eyes," created by bacteria during the fermentation process. Swiss Cheese without eyes is known as "blind."

The terms Swiss or Baby Swiss are also applied to cheeses of this style made outside Switzerland, such as Jarlsberg Cheese which originated in Norway.
In general, the larger the eyes in a Swiss Cheese, the more pronounced its flavor because of a longer fermentation period which gives the bacteria more time to act. This can pose a problem, however, because cheese with large eyes do not slice well and can come apart in mechanical slicers. As a result, industry regulators have limited the eye size by which Swiss Cheese receives the Grand A stamp.

Talleggio

Taleggio is a popular cheese that originated in Italy. With 48 percent fat, it is one of the earliest sponge-like cheeses. The cheese is aged for almost ten weeks, and to ensure that it is fungus-free, it is washed every week with seawater. Though the piquant smell might put you off, at first, Taleggio is, in fact, quite delicious with a subtle, fruity taste and tastes best when served as a side with Italian Nebbiolo wine.

Recommended Reading

There are so many wonderful books available to inspire you and increase your party and entertaining skills!

How to Win Friends and Influence People by Dale Carnegie

Barefoot Contessa Parties by Ina Garten

Entertaining at Home by R. Carman

Celebrate Everything! by Darcy Miller

The Unqualified Hostess by Whoopi Goldberg

Life is a Party by David Burke

Batch Cocktails by Maggie Hoffman

Southern Entertainers Cookbook by Courtney Whitmore

Charcuterie Boards by Marco Nicoli

About the Author

For the past several years, Chris Cooper has delighted in teaching several Lifestyle classes through The Enrichment Academy in the Villages, Florida. One of her popular classes, "Entertaining with Grace and Style" was the inspiration for this book along with the urging of her enthusiastic students. One of the primary goals of her classes is to share her secrets and techniques for stress-free entertaining to enjoy one's own fabulous party.

After Chris earned her degree in Interior Design, she joined her mother's growing catering business in the San Francisco Bay area. The catering business was her mother's passion and continued to grow until her retirement. Ethel Cooper's systems and techniques along with Chris' design and presentation skills made for a successful event planning partnership.

Chris went on to earn her real estate license and utilized her event planning skills to elevate the marketing of her homes for sale listings. Her last position as Vice President and Director of Training for Prudential allowed her to share successful event planning and marketing techniques with her students.

Chris became a pioneer in Home Staging after recognizing the need for this special marketing support in the real estate industry. Her eye for design and presentation skills caused her business to expand quickly to eighteen employees, five trucks, and four warehouses full of furniture. Chris personally staged more than 3000 homes over her twenty years of experience and earned her numerous awards including Professional Home Stager of the Year.

Chris also completed beautiful interior design projects for residential and commercial spaces including international projects. She has been a member of numerous Interior Design and Home Staging organizations including Real Estate Staging Association Pro, Certified Staging and Redesign Professional, Association of Staging Professionals, and International Association of Staging Professionals, and ASID.

Recognized as a Master in Home Staging, Chris was an invited guest lecturer at Stanford University for five years on the value of Home Staging in Real Estate Investing. Through teaching, Chris found energy and satisfaction in passing along her years of experience and valuable tips. Along with teaching classes at The Enrichment Academy, in The Villages, Florida, Chris has also been a speaker at various conventions and is a certified speaker on the subject of Home Staging for the State of Florida Department of Real Estate.

    Chris Cooper's unique blend of Event planning, entertaining, interior design, and presentation talents qualifies her to be a Lifestyle Expert sharing her ideas for living with grace and style!

To inquire about Chris speaking to your group or for interviews:

Email: chriscooper@yahoo.com
Website: www.chriscooperdesign.com

www.ingramcontent.com/pod-product-compliance
Lightning Source LLC
Chambersburg PA
CBHW062004060526
44119CB00110B/161